Women's Health
Today 2001

Women's Health Today 2001

The Latest Breakthroughs for the Female Body

from the Editors of *Prevention* Magazine

RODALE

© 2001 by Rodale Inc.

Prevention is a registered trademark of Rodale Inc.

Printed in the United States of America
Rodale Inc. makes every effort to use acid-free ∞, recycled paper ♻ .

ISBN 1–57954–358–8 hardcover
ISBN 1–57954–394–4 paperback

Distributed to the book trade by St. Martin's Press

2   4   6   8   10   9   7   5   3   1   hardcover
2   4   6   8   10   9   7   5   3   1   paperback

Visit us on the Web at www.preventionbookshelf.com, or call us toll-free at (800) 848-4735.

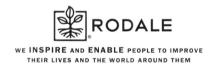

WE **INSPIRE** AND **ENABLE** PEOPLE TO IMPROVE
THEIR LIVES AND THE WORLD AROUND THEM

Women's Health Today 2001 Staff

EDITOR: Diane Gardiner Kozak

WRITERS: Maureen Boland, Karen Cicero, Bridget Doherty, Toby Hanlon, Ed.D., Marjorie Ingall, Joely Johnson, Madeline Johnson, Danielle Kost, Diane Kozak, Barbara Loecher, Gale Maleskey, Holly McCord, R.D., Susan McQuillan, R.D., Gloria McVeigh, Jeff Meade, Mary Jane Minkin, Melinda Minton, Linda Mooney, Kristine Napier, R.D., M.P.H., Colleen Pierre, R.D., Linda Rao, Sarah Robertson, Martha Schindler, Susan C. Smith, Maggie Spilner, Michele Stanten, Julia VanTine, Zachary Veilleux, Teri Walsh, Denise Webb, Selene Yeager

ASSOCIATE ART DIRECTOR: Richard Kershner

INTERIOR DESIGNER: Richard Kershner

COVER DESIGNER: Christopher Rhoads

PHOTO EDITOR: James A. Gallucci

ASSISTANT RESEARCH MANAGER: Shea Zukowski

PRIMARY RESEARCH EDITOR: Anita C. Small

RESEARCH EDITORS: Carol J. Gilmore, Jennifer Bright

DEVELOPMENTAL EDITOR: Amy K. Kovalski

COPY EDITOR: Kelly L. Schmidt

EDITORIAL PRODUCTION MANAGER: Marilyn Hauptly

LAYOUT DESIGNER: Daniel MacBride

MANUFACTURING COORDINATORS: Brenda Miller, Jodi Schaffer, Patrick T. Smith

Rodale Healthy Living Books

EDITOR IN CHIEF, *PREVENTION*: Catherine Cassidy

EXECUTIVE EDITOR: Tammerly Booth

DIRECTOR OF SERIES DEVELOPMENT: Gary Krebs

EDITORIAL DIRECTOR: Michael Ward

VICE PRESIDENT AND MARKETING DIRECTOR: Karen Arbegast

PRODUCT MARKETING DIRECTOR: Guy Maake

BOOK MANUFACTURING DIRECTOR: Helen Clogston

MANUFACTURING MANAGER: Eileen Bauder

RESEARCH DIRECTOR: Ann Gossy Yermish

COPY MANAGER: Lisa D. Andruscavage

PRODUCTION MANAGER: Robert V. Anderson Jr.

DIGITAL PROCESSING GROUP ASSOCIATE MANAGER: Thomas P. Aczel

OFFICE MANAGER: Jacqueline Dornblaser

OFFICE STAFF: Susan B. Dorschutz, Julie Kehs Minnix, Tara Schrantz, Catherine E. Strouse

Board of Advisors

Rosemary Agostini, M.D. Primary care sports medicine physician at the Virginia Mason Sports Medicine Center and clinical associate professor of orthopedics at the University of Washington, both in Seattle

Barbara D. Bartlik, M.D. Clinical assistant professor in the department of psychiatry at Weill Medical College of Cornell University and assistant attending psychiatrist at the New York–Presbyterian Hospital, both in New York City

Mary Ruth Buchness, M.D. Chief of dermatology at St. Vincent's Hospital and Medical Center in New York City and associate professor of dermatology and medicine at the New York Medical College in Valhalla

Leah J. Dickstein, M.D. Professor and associate chair for academic affairs in the department of psychiatry and behavioral sciences and associate dean for faculty and student advocacy at the University of Louisville School of Medicine in Kentucky and past president of the American Medical Women's Association (AMWA)

Jean L. Fourcroy, M.D., Ph.D. Past president of the American Medical Women's Association (AMWA) and of the National Council on Women's Health

JoAnn E. Manson, M.D., Dr.P.H. Professor of medicine at Harvard Medical School and chief of preventive medicine at Brigham and Women's Hospital in Boston

Susan C. Olson, Ph.D. Clinical psychologist, life transition/psychospiritual therapist, and weight-management consultant in Seattle

Mary Lake Polan, M.D., Ph.D. Professor and chair of the department of gynecology and obstetrics at Stanford University School of Medicine

Lila Amdurska Wallis, M.D., M.A.C.P. Clinical professor of medicine at Weill Medical College of Cornell University in New York City, past president of the American Medical Women's Association (AMWA), founding president of the National Council on Women's Health, director of continuing medical education programs for physicians, and master and laureate of the American College of Physicians

Carla Wolper, R.D. Nutritionist and clinical coordinator at the obesity research center at St. Luke's–Roosevelt Hospital Center and nutritionist at the center for women's health at Columbia-Presbyterian/Eastside, both in New York City

CONTENTS

LIFESTYLE RESTYLE

When a New Jersey woman learned dieting was about her brain, not her stomach, she had a "midlife miracle."

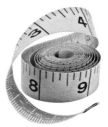

Measure Your Risk: Why abdominal size matters
PAGE 6

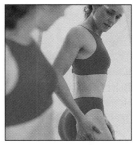

Cellulite Solutions: Can massage do more than relax you?
PAGE 28

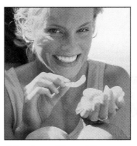

Olestra: The skinny on fake fat
PAGE 42

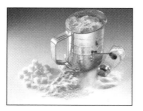

A White Lie:
Learn the truth
behind a diet
PAGE 56

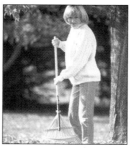

Burning Questions:
How long does it take
to use an additional
150 calories?
PAGE 97

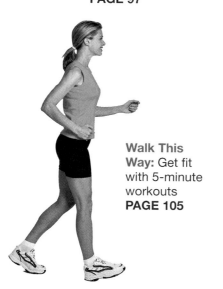

**Walk This
Way:** Get fit
with 5-minute
workouts
PAGE 105

LIFESTYLE RESTYLE

PART THREE
Fitting In Fitness

LIFESTYLE RESTYLE

PART FOUR

Disease Defense for the Female Body

LIFESTYLE RESTYLE

PART FIVE

Relax Your Mind, Rejuvenate Your Soul

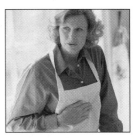

Read the Signs: Women's heart attack symptoms may differ from men's
PAGE 137

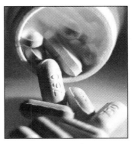

Niacin: Supplement your efforts to lower cholesterol
PAGE 153

Give Cancer the Slip: Physical activity can lower your risk
PAGE 173

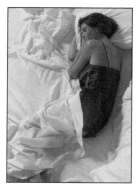

Sleep Secrets:
What your mind does
after dark
PAGE 198

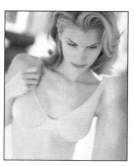

A Good Foundation:
Choose the right bra
to look your best
PAGE 214

PART SIX

Age Erasers
for Real Women

Introduction

This Is the Year You Finally Lose Weight

If you're like me, the past year has been super-busy with work, with family and friends, with classes . . . you name it. In the craziness of it all, what did you and I do for ourselves? What choices did we make to ensure that we enjoy many more happy, healthy, crazy years like this one?

Choice is largely what our good health is all about. As you read through the pages of *Women's Health Today 2001,* you'll find hundreds of ideas 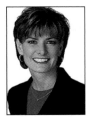 for things you can choose to start doing today, *right now,* to move yourself toward better health. Health isn't built in huge leaps and bounds, but by little "deposits" made over the course of your lifetime. This book is devoted to some of the most important small things (and some not so small things) you can do to make a very big difference.

One of the best choices you can make for yourself is to finally lose unwanted pounds—and keep them off. Did you know that shrinking your belly helps lower cholesterol? You'll find the 9 easy steps in this book. You'll also find 25 solutions to 6 of the most common weight-loss dilemmas. And forget calorie counting! We all hate it. Learn the 5 incredibly simple strategies for cutting and burning calories to make a significant difference in your waistline.

Another one of the smart choices you can make this year is to get moving. Studies show that only about one-quarter of American women get 30 minutes of exercise a day! But you can incorporate exercise into your day easily and without the hassles of going to the gym. Everything counts, from raking the leaves and vacuuming the rugs to playing tag with your kids. You'll find dozens of new ways to expend more energy within the course of your normal daily routine that will add up to real weight loss.

In the pages that follow, you'll find all the information you need to make the right choices to live a healthier and happier. You'll discover what the latest medical and scientific research means to you, and learn simple steps that help with everything from dealing with cravings to detecting signs of heart disease. With sections on heart attack, cholesterol, osteoporosis, diabetes, cancer, relaxation, and skin care and teeth, this book provides you with everything you need to know about early warning signs, preventive and diagnostic testing, and treatment.

You have to give your body what it needs, no matter what the latest fad or trend dictates. Remember that if you do right by your body, it will do right by you. So keep this book handy, and use it in good health!

Catherine M. Cassidy

Catherine Cassidy
Editor in Chief
Prevention Magazine

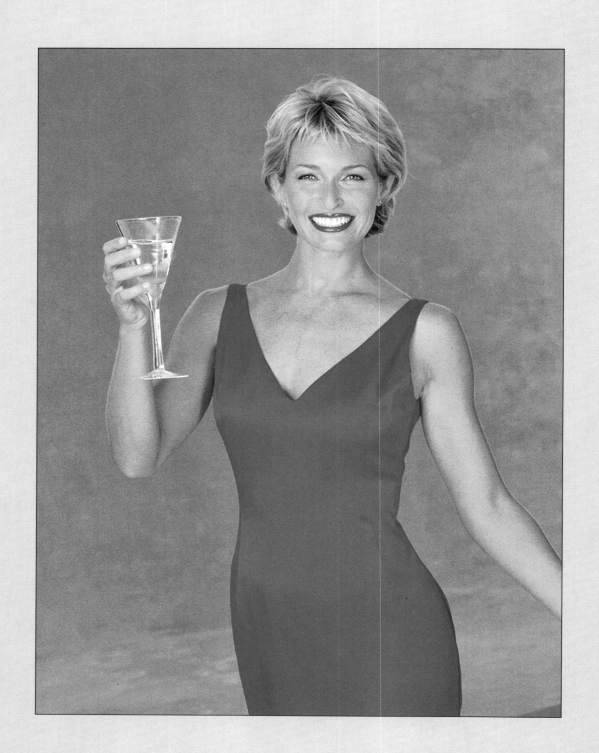

Part One

Lose
All the Weight
You Want

Chapter 1

Minimize Your Middle, Maximize Your Health

Nine simple ways to take off inches for benefits beyond your waistband.

You're way past worrying about having a waist size the likes of which only Barbie knows. If you do keep tabs on your measurements, it's most likely to help you get the right fit when you order clothing from catalogs.

When it comes to your health, however, there's one simple measurement that can protect you in some very big ways, even if you're not overweight. Studies show that a waistline of 32 inches (37 inches for men) or more may put you at greater risk for health problems.

Unlike fat on your thighs—which may bug you, but doesn't pose much of a health risk— the size of your belly is directly related to your risk of disease. Scientific research continues to demonstrate that a trim middle can protect you against life-threatening diseases such as breast cancer, heart disease, diabetes, and more.

Get More Than a Slim Silhouette

A flat belly does more than make you look fit and sexy; it can actually save your life. Fat inside the abdomen is more likely to release fatty acids into the liver than fat elsewhere on the body, says Henry S. Kahn, M.D., associate professor of family and preventive medicine at Emory University School of Medicine in Atlanta. The result can be excessive amounts of cholesterol and insulin in the bloodstream, plus altered hormone levels, all of which play a role in the development of disease. But you don't have to let that happen. Here are some of the things you can achieve by reducing your waistline.

Dodge diabetes. Women with the highest waist circumferences—36 inches or larger—were five times more likely to develop diabetes, compared to those whose waistlines

HealthPoint

Lose Weight, Not Your Gallbladder

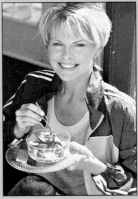

Your chances of needing your gallbladder removed are more than three times higher if you're overweight. But you may also be at risk if you lose and regain weight again and again.

A recent study of more than 47,000 women showed that those with the highest body mass indexes (BMI)—30 to 35—were at this triple risk compared with women with lower BMIs. And women who regained more than 20 pounds during a 16-year period were 1½ times more likely to need gallbladder surgery than those who maintained their weight loss.

But don't give up trying to achieve a slim figure. "Instead, lose weight gradually," says study coauthor Eugenie H. Coakley of Brigham and Women's Hospital in Boston.

Aim to lose no more than 1 to 2 pounds a week. You can do that by eating 200 fewer calories (about two slices of cheese) and exercising off another 300 calories (about an hour-long walk) each day.

To calculate your BMI, divide your weight (in pounds) by your height (in inches) squared, then multiply that total by 705. So if you are a 5-foot-5-inch woman who weighs 140 pounds, you will divide 140 by 4225 (65 inches × 65 inches) and then multiply the result (.033) by 705 to get a BMI of 23. Anything over 25 is considered overweight.

measured in at about 26 inches, according to the landmark Nurses' Health Study of more than 43,000 women. "Abdominal fat appears to be related to insulin resistance," says Dr. Kahn. That means that your cells don't respond to insulin as they should. As a result, your blood sugar levels remain unusually high. It's likely that over time, this resistance causes your body to stop producing insulin, resulting in middle-

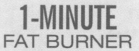

1-MINUTE FAT BURNER

Schedule a blood test. About 1 in every 12 women (most of whom don't know it) has an underactive thyroid, which can slow down her metabolism.

age diabetes. "Insulin resistance may also help create yet more abdominal fat," he explains.

Avoid a heart attack. When researchers tracked more than 44,000 women for 8 years, they found that those who had waists larger than 32 inches had more than double the risk of having a heart attack than their slimmer counterparts. That's no surprise when you consider that women with waists more than 32 inches are also more likely to have major risk factors: They're nearly 50 percent more likely

to have high cholesterol and close to 60 percent more likely to have high blood pressure than their leaner peers. And those same fatty deposits that clog arteries and lead to heart attacks can also clog arteries that feed the brain, putting you at higher risk for a stroke.

Prevent breast cancer. Another disadvantage of abdominal fat may be its effect on hormone levels. "Postmenopausal women with central fat patterns tend to have unbalanced levels of hormones, and that may be why they have higher rates of breast cancer," says Jacob Seidell, Ph.D., of the National Institute of Public Health in Bilthoven, Netherlands. In one study, women with breast cancer had an average of 45 percent more abdominal fat than healthy women. Endometrial cancer is also two to three times more common in overweight women than in those who are lean.

Lower your blood pressure. People who are overweight are more prone to high blood pressure, a risk factor for stroke and heart attack, says Jan I. Maby, D.O., director of the geriatric medical home care program at Mount Sinai Medical Center in New York City. Every pound of excess weight drives your systolic blood pressure (the top number in a blood pressure reading) up 4.5 millimeters.

Beat back pain. Women with larger

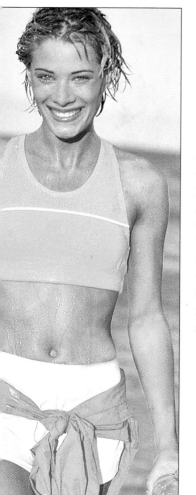

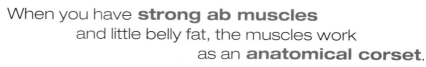

When you have **strong ab muscles** and little belly fat, the muscles work as an **anatomical corset**.

waists have 20 to 50 percent more back problems than women with narrower waists. "When you have strong ab muscles and little belly fat, the muscles work as an anatomical corset, strengthening your ability to support your upper body, improving posture, and relieving pressure on your back," says Len Kravitz, Ph.D., graduate coordinator of wellness at the University of Mississippi in Oxford.

Breathe easier. Although your body can keep getting bigger, your lungs can't. The same two lungs that did so well when you were thinner now have to supply oxygen to a larger body. That puts a lot of strain on your respiratory system, Dr. Maby says. Belly fat can actually crowd organs, creating breathing difficulties. Even moderate amounts of abdominal fat can make you more prone to wheezing, coughing, and shortness of breath. It also increases the likelihood of sleep apnea, a condition associated with stroke, high blood pressure, and heart attack.

Boost your circulation. Excess weight, especially in the abdomen, presses on the veins in the upper thighs and groin, causing them to weaken. Circulation slows, resulting in

Stay Slim during Menopause

The average woman gains 2 to 5 pounds at menopause, but it's not uncommon for some women to gain as much as 30 pounds—most of it in the belly. "The drop-off in estrogen at menopause seems to have a permissive effect on fat accumulation in the abdomen, while actually blocking accumulation in the hips and thighs," says Jennifer C. Lovejoy, Ph.D., chief of the women's nutrition research program at Louisiana State University in Baton Rouge. But weight gain at menopause is not inevitable. Here are some extra steps to maintain a happy middle.

- Pay more attention to diet and exercise. One study from the University of Vermont in Burlington followed women through menopause and found that they ate an extra 150 calories a day on average, while reducing physical activity by 150 calories a day. "Decreasing levels of estrogen may result in an increased preference for fats and sweets," notes Dr. Lovejoy. To counteract this effect, keep track of how much you're eating and exercising.

- Ask about replacement therapy. Research shows that women who opt for hormone-replacement therapy (HRT) during menopause are less likely to accumulate belly fat. "I'd hate to see anybody make the decision about hormone replacement solely because of this, but it is something to factor into the decision," says Dr. Lovejoy. Talk to your doctor about whether HRT is right for you.

increased pressure in the veins. The result: varicose veins. If you are more than 15 percent over your ideal weight, chances are that the excess pounds are putting stress on your veins in one way or another, says J. A. Olivencia, M.D., vascular surgeon and medical director of the Iowa Vein Center in West Des Moines, Iowa. "When people are overweight, they become less active. Their clothing will be tight and constrict blood-flow." That constriction only makes varicose veins worse.

Ease up on your joints. Excess weight causes greater wear and tear on joints and can aggravate symptoms of arthritis. The strain is particularly hard on your knees and lower back.

Nine Easy Steps to Shrink Your Belly

We scoured the latest scientific research and talked to leading experts to find out the best ways to get your tummy in line. Here are nine lifestyle strategies that can help take inches from your waistline—and make you healthier all over.

1. Eat like a Vegetarian

The best way to predict whether or not you'll need larger pants is to look at your plate. In a 10-year study of nearly 80,000 people, "women who ate the most meat (more than seven servings a week) were 1½ times more likely to expand their waistlines than were women who

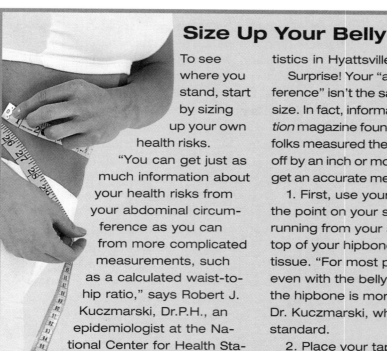

Size Up Your Belly

To see where you stand, start by sizing up your own health risks.

"You can get just as much information about your health risks from your abdominal circumference as you can from more complicated measurements, such as a calculated waist-to-hip ratio," says Robert J. Kuczmarski, Dr.P.H., an epidemiologist at the National Center for Health Statistics in Hyattsville, Maryland.

Surprise! Your "abdominal circumference" isn't the same as your waist size. In fact, informal tests at *Prevention* magazine found that when most folks measured their waists, they were off by an inch or more. Here's how to get an accurate measurement.

1. First, use your thumb to feel for the point on your side (think of a line running from your armpit) where the top of your hipbone gives way to soft tissue. "For most people, this point is even with the belly button, but using the hipbone is more reliable," says Dr. Kuczmarski, who developed the standard.

2. Place your tape measure just

ate two servings or less," says Dr. Kahn.

This doesn't mean that you have to give up meat. It's about moderation. "Few people in our study were vegetarians," Dr. Kahn says. "They just ate like they were." Limit yourself to one serving of meat every 2 to 3 days, and make up the difference with fruits and veggies—at least five servings a day. "They act as 'protection' against gaining weight."

2. Eat Early, Eat Often

Many dieters develop the unfortunate habit of skipping meals, getting most of the day's calories from just one or two large meals, one of which is usually in the evening. That's trouble. Studies have shown that people who spread their food intake over the course of the day take in fewer calories overall and tend to eat more healthful foods (presumably because their snack choices aren't driven by hunger). The best plan: Eat five or six small meals throughout the day.

3. Walk Every Day

No matter how much you change your diet, abdominal fat isn't going anywhere unless you get up and move. Specifically, it requires aerobic exercise. "As you decrease overall body fat, you'll end up with a leaner waistline," says Kathryn M. Rexrode, M.D., associate physician and instructor in the division of preventive medicine at Harvard Medical School.

Walking is among the best forms of exercise to keep belly fat in check. Dr. Kahn's study found that women who walked regularly were 16 percent less likely to gain inches at the waist than those who didn't. "There's a major, consistent effect from walking, but you need to walk 4 hours a week, or at least 30 minutes every day, to see it," he says.

4. Tone Your Tummy

"Thin may sound good, but when it comes to abs, toned is what you really want. Thin people can end up with Pillsbury Doughboy tummies if they don't train their ab muscles specifically," says Dr. Kravitz. "Even though they're thin, they're flabby." Ab-strengthening exercises are the key to getting a belly worth baring. Strong ab muscles also help protect your back.

5. Build Muscle

"Resistance training is an important component of a belly-slimming workout because it increases muscle mass throughout the body, helping to boost metabolism," says Dr. Kravitz.

above that bone, and loop it around your belly, being careful to keep it parallel to the floor. Use a full-length mirror to be sure.

3. Breathe normally while you read the result. Don't cheat by putting extra tension on the tape!

A waistline of more than 32 inches (37 inches for men) may put you at a higher risk for health problems. Anything more than 35 inches (40 inches for men) is serious cause for concern, according to guidelines from the National Institutes of Health. "That's the level at which your risk of diabetes, high blood pressure, and heart disease rises considerably," cautions Dr. Kuczmarski.

Know at a Glance Where You Stand

Find your height on the chart to the right. Follow the line upward to see in which zone your weight falls, then read the consequences below.

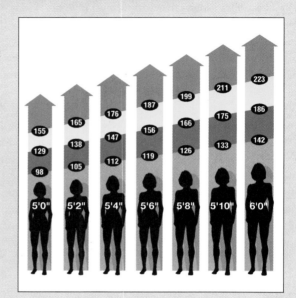

Red Zone: Alert!

Your weight is putting you at ultrahigh risk for chronic diseases. Four out of five people in this range have diabetes, high cholesterol levels, high blood pressure, heart disease, gallbladder disease, or osteoarthritis. And 40 percent have two or more of these ailments.

Yellow Zone: Caution!

Your enjoyment of life will start to be impacted by excess pounds. Nonsmoking yellow-zoners, for instance, have as much trouble walking uphill as pack-a-day smokers. You'll start to see a rise in rates of diseases such as diabetes and hypertension, with more illness the higher up the scale you go.

Green Zone: Congratulations!

Your weight enhances your chances of living a long, vigorous life. But don't let your guard down—maintaining healthy weight takes a lifelong commitment.

The more muscle you develop, whether in your arms, shoulders, or back, the greater your ability to burn calories before your body can turn them into fat. In addition, building upper-body muscles, such as in your arms and shoulders, can make your waistline look smaller. For a total-body workout, see Trade Fat for Muscle in 10 Minutes a Day on page 108.

6. Take Vitamin E

Experts have been recommending vitamin E supplements for years to protect you from heart attacks, colds and flu, cancer, diabetes, and Alzheimer's disease. Now there is preliminary evidence that vitamin E may be a potential fat-fighter, too. "It may help prevent abdominal weight gain by protecting against insulin resistance," says Dr. Kahn. Aim for 100 to 400 IU a day.

7. Adjust Your Attitude

Crank up the Mozart, take a walk, get a massage, talk to a friend, breathe deeply—do anything that keeps you calm. Studies have shown that women who don't control their stress tend to have larger waistlines. The culprit appears to be cortisol, which is a hormone released by the body during periods of stress. It's believed that increased cortisol levels play a role in directing fat to the abdominal area.

8. Enjoy Your Friends

Having a workout buddy is a great way to help you stick to your fitness regimen. But some experts suggest that buddies—even those you don't work out with—can help you meet your workout goals. Those people who reported the most social support from spouses, family, and friends were the least likely to gain weight during a 3-year study. Researchers say that a wide social network may help reduce stress, improve self-esteem, and encourage better health practices.

9. Cut Out the Cocktails

Dr. Kahn's study also found that women who drank beer or liquor one to four times a week were more likely to put on abdominal inches than women who didn't. If you do drink, stick to wine, which was not associated with waist gain and may offer heart-protective effects that beer and liquor may not.

1-MINUTE FAT BURNER

Drink, drink, drink. Dehydration can slow your metabolism by 3 percent. If you weigh 150 pounds, that's about 45 fewer calories burned a day. That could add up to 5 pounds a year.

Chapter 2

Calories Count, but You Don't Have To

Five no-math strategies to make the weight-loss equation work for you.

No matter what weight-loss plan you choose, the bottom line is still this: "If you take in more calories than you burn, you'll gain weight. End of story," says Louis Martin, M.D., medical director of the Louisiana State University Weight Management Center in New Orleans.

Need further proof that calories count? Ponder these sobering statistics.

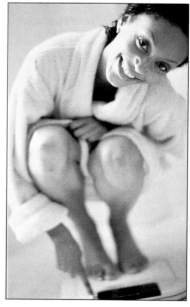

• In 1978, the average woman consumed 1,571 calories a day. Today, she takes in about 1,710 calories. That measly 139-calorie difference translates to 14 extra pounds a year.

• We consume less fat than ever before (33 percent of our total calories, down from 40 percent in 1978), yet a record 50 million of us are overweight.

• Less than 40 percent of us get regular exercise, the world's best calorie-burner.

The upshot: You can run from calories, but you can't hide, because they'll hunt you down, grab on to your hips, and cling for dear life.

Fortunately, you can fight back. Your reward: a slimmer, healthier body and jeans you can breathe in.

Maximum Nutrition, Minimum Calories

Counting calories has all the appeal of a a tax audit. So it's a good thing that the latest word from nutritionists is "don't bother."

"Unless you want to eat with a calculator in hand, there's no need to count calories," says Lisa Tartamella, R.D., a registered dietitian and ambulatory nutrition specialist at the Centers of Nutrition, Yale–New Haven Hospital in Connecticut.

The alternative: Eat mindfully. And that boils down to certain basics: Become aware of portion sizes. Shed your "supersize it" mindset. Cut back on fat. Monitor your intake of low-fat snacks and sweets, which can be treacherously high in calories.

And yes, go ahead and splurge on your favorite foods now and then. Because life without ice cream, buffalo wings, and sausage sandwiches would be bleak indeed.

For the most part, though, mindful eating should be nutritious eating. "The goal is to get maximum nutrition with minimum calories," explains Franca Alphin, R.D., a registered dietitian and administrative director of the Duke University Diet and Fitness Center in Durham, North Carolina. That means eating more low-calorie, health-enhancing fruits, vegetables, whole grains, and beans. And consuming less

Where Have All Your Calories Gone?

Assuming you don't take in more calories than you need, here's how your body uses what you give it.

• Basal metabolism. From 60 to 65 percent of your calories are spent just keeping you alive and kicking—keeping your heart beating, your kidneys filtering waste, and your temperature hovering near 98 degrees.

• Physical activity. Another 25 percent goes to pure movement, from running up and down the field during your kid's soccer game to working up a sweat in step class.

• Thermic effect of food. The remaining 10 percent of calories is spent processing food. (Yes, it takes calories to process calories!)

sugary, fatty fare, which is calorie-dense and nutrient-poor.

But it's not enough to curtail calories. You need to burn them, too.

Ready to achieve a higher state of calorie consciousness? Here's a (virtually) calculator-free guide to calories—how many you need to maintain or lose weight, how to whittle the excess calories from your diet, and how to crank up your calorie-burning power.

HealthPoint

Lose Weight—Not Brainpower

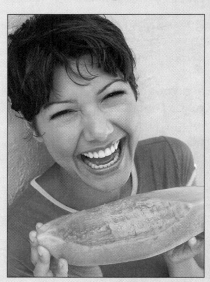

Eating too few calories a day may lower your iron levels and impair your concentration. When 14 obese, premenopausal women were put on diets of 1,000 to 1,200 calories (half of what they usually ate) for 15 weeks, seven of the women's iron levels dropped—despite the fact that they were getting about twice the recommended amount of iron. These women also scored 50 percent lower on a concentration test than women with adequate levels of iron.

"Our bodies may not use iron as effectively when we restrict calories," says study author Mary Kretsch, Ph.D., of the USDA Agricultural Research Service in San Francisco.

So how can you lower the number on your scale without also lowering your iron status?

Eat at least 1,200 calories a day. Fewer than that could not only lower your iron level but also slow your metabolism—and your weight loss progress.

Get tested. A blood test that measures hemoglobin and serum ferritin levels will tell you if your iron levels are low.

Do not take iron supplements unless recommended by a doctor. Some research suggests that too much iron may raise the risk of heart disease and colon cancer.

Stock up before dieting. "Get extra iron to build up your reserves before starting a reduced-calorie diet," Dr. Kretsch advises. Good sources include lean meats; beans; broccoli; kale; and iron-enriched breads, pasta, rice, and cereal.

How Many Calories Do You Need?

Your calorie needs depend on your resting metabolism, which is influenced by your height, weight, age, gender, activity level, and ratio of muscle to fat, among other variables, says Carmen Conrey, R.D., clinical dietitian specialist at the Johns Hopkins Weight Management Center in Baltimore.

Tall, big-boned women typically need more calories than petite women. Active women need more calories than sedentary ones. And, oddly, those of us who are packing a few more pounds than we'd like need more calories than those of us who are at a desirable weight. (It takes more energy to power a larger body.)

Still, without taking muscle-to-fat ratios into account, you can get a down-and-dirty estimate of your individual calorie needs with a few strokes of the calculator.

Divide your current weight by 2.2 in order to convert pounds to kilograms. Then multiply your weight in kilograms by 30, which is the number of calories you need per pound of body weight.

So if you're 150 pounds, you weigh 68 kilograms. Multiply 68 by 30 and you arrive at 2,040 calories, the amount you need to maintain that weight. If your body mass index is 30 or higher, or you are about 30 pounds overweight, however, this calculation may overestimate your calorie requirements because body fat does not require as many calories as muscle.

To lose weight, multiply your weight in kilograms by 25. In the example above, to lose about 1½ pounds a week, you would need to consume 1,700 calories a day. That's 340 fewer calories than the calorie requirement to maintain your weight.

Once you've done the math, you'll see how shaving a few hundred calories from your diet can make a significant difference in your waistline. And it's incredibly simple to do. These calorie-trimming strategies can help.

1. Go on Portion Patrol

To trim your calorie budget, you need to trim your portion sizes, says Alphin. But that's not always easy in America, Land of the Free and Home of the Supersized Portion.

Many restaurants—especially our favorite chains—serve bowls of pasta as deep as a 10-gallon hat, steaks half the size of a Frisbee, and muffins as big as grapefruits. A popular pizza chain actually had to design a new box and cutting board for one of their most calorie-dense pizzas.

"It's absolutely unbelievable how restaurant portion sizes have changed over the years," says Alphin. "But restaurants aren't entirely to blame. We're not satisfied unless we're served meals that hang over the plate."

And boy, do they hang. When nutritionists from the Center for Science in the Public Interest (CSPI) in Washington, D.C., compared restaurant portions of 18 foods with the government's "official" serving sizes, here's a sampling of what they found.

• The government says a tuna salad sandwich weighs 4 ounces and contains 340 calories. A typical restaurant tuna

The goal is maximum nutrition with minimum calories.

What We Really Eat

The now familiar food pyramid at left is a visual guide to what the United States Department of Agriculture considers the ideal American diet. The lop-sided pyramid at right shows what the average person was actually eating in 1996, the latest year studied.

The most striking difference? The bulge at the top of the what-we-really-eat pyramid representing fats, oils, and sweets.

To see how your own eating habits measure up, check out the USDA Inter-active Healthy Eating Index. The Web site, www.usda.gov/cnpp, analyzes specific foods and rates them according to nutritional content. With the help of this free, interactive tool, Internet users can gauge their diets and maintain a cumulative record to observe their progress.

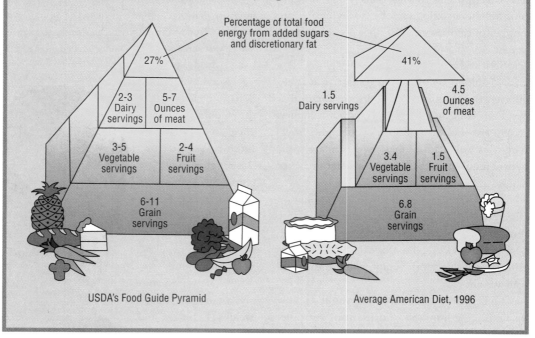

Percentage of total food energy from added sugars and discretionary fat

27%

2-3 Dairy servings | 5-7 Ounces of meat

3-5 Vegetable servings | 2-4 Fruit servings

6-11 Grain servings

USDA's Food Guide Pyramid

41%

1.5 Dairy servings | 4.5 Ounces of meat

3.4 Vegetable servings | 1.5 Fruit servings

6.8 Grain servings

Average American Diet, 1996

sandwich weighs more than 10 ounces and contains 720 calories.

• Officially, a serving of french fries is 3 ounces and 220 calories. A McDonald's Super Size Fries: 6 ounces, 540 calories.

• A standard 3-cup serving of unbuttered popcorn has 160 calories. A small movie-theater tub of unbuttered popcorn has 7 cups and 400 calories; a medium, 16 cups and 900 calories.

"In fact, at one of the leading fast-food chains,

the hamburger found in the kid's meals used to be the only adult-size portion available," says Jayne Hurley, R.D., a registered dietitian and the senior nutritionist at CSPI who co-led the study.

We help ourselves to plus-size portions at home, too. Who among us hasn't eaten half a bag of chips at one sitting or gone back for seconds (and maybe thirds) on meat loaf and mashed potatoes?

"In my view, huge portion sizes and inactivity are the reasons one out of three Americans are overweight," says Tartamella. "When I show women what one serving of pasta or mashed potatoes actually looks like, they're absolutely astonished."

As obvious as it sounds, we need to start paying attention to the serving size portion of food labels, says Alphin. For example, more often than not, the bottled fruit juice or the bag of chips you have with lunch contains 2 or $2\frac{1}{2}$ servings rather than 1.

Second, practice calorie visualization. "Learn what one serving of a particular food really looks like," says Alphin. For example, one serving of meat is 3 ounces and fits in the palm of your hand; one serving of pasta is $\frac{1}{2}$ cup and the size of a scoop of ice cream. See "Visualize Those Calories" on page 16 for more ways to eyeball portion sizes.

The tips below can help streamline serving sizes, at home or on the go.

• Keep food on the stove or counter rather than on the table. Those few extra seconds it takes to get off your chair for another plateful will remind you to pass up a second serving.

• If you normally eat 2 to 3 cups of pasta (400 to 600 calories) at one sitting, "stretch" 1 cup (200 calories) with a cup of grilled or sautéed veggies.

The 10 Most Satisfying Foods

Researchers in Australia have actually identified the foods most likely to quell hunger pangs. The top 10: potatoes, fish, oatmeal, oranges, apples, whole wheat pasta, beefsteak, grapes, air-popped popcorn, and bran cereal.

• Instead of toting a whole box of cookies or a whole bag of chips to the TV, measure out one serving and put it on a plate.

• Dilute fruit juice with water. One serving of cranberry juice is 6 ounces and 108 calories. But bottles of fruit juice routinely contain 16 ounces. Drink that much and you've just swallowed 288 calories. If you dilute it with water by half and drink 8 ounces instead of 16, you'll consume a more sensible 72 calories.

• When you order pizza, eat one or two slices, rather than three or four.

• At fast-food restaurants, order à la carte rather than being lured by the "combo packages" of large burger, large fries, and large drink.

2. Avoid "Low-Fat Syndrome"

It's just another story of love and betrayal. The low-fat or fat-free cookies, pastries, and chips we've grown to love seduce us with their healthy promises—but then blow our calorie budget out of the water.

Truth is, many low-fat products contain as many calories as their full-fat counterparts.

• A low-fat apple-cinnamon Pop Tart contains 191 calories; its full-fat counterpart, 200 calories.

• A fat-free Apple Newton contains about 50 calories. So does a regular Fig Newton.

• An ounce of regular cheese curls has 150 calories. The reduced-fat kind, 130 calories.

Don't blame the cookiemakers. They print the appropriate serving size and its calorie content right on the Nutrition Facts label. "But somehow, our brains interpret 'fat-free' or 'low-fat' as 'calorie-free,'" says Alphin. "So we tend to eat huge portions of low-fat foods, which can double or even triple our calorie intake."

The antidote? Once again, portion control. Try these suggestions.

• Look for single-portion low-fat or fat-free snacks, readily available at convenience stores.

• If you buy low-fat snacks by the box or bag, divide them into one-serving portions and store in plastic bags.

• Store boxes of low-fat pastry, snack cakes, or doughnuts in the back of your highest kitchen cabinet. When you want some, measure out one serving and immediately stash the rest away again.

• Consume a small amount of protein (perhaps a glass of skim milk) with your low-fat snacks. "The protein will help you feel a little more satisfied," explains Conrey.

3. Eat Food with Heft

Try this sometime. Measure out 3 cups of strawberries. Then put them next to 10 large jelly beans.

Both contain about 100 calories. What's dramatically different is the *amount* of food you get for those calories.

This powerful visual is a perfect demonstration of energy density, or how many calories a food packs for a given weight.

Strawberries—along with other fruits, vegetables, and many grains—have a low energy density, which means you can eat more of the

---

Visualize Those Calories

To most of us, "one portion" is whatever our appetite tells us it is. But being unaware of real-world portion size is the main cause of climbing calorie intakes—and widening hips. Here's how to eyeball one portion with the precision of a Wild West sharpshooter.

• 3 ounces of meat: the size of a cassette tape

• 3 ounces of grilled fish: the size of your checkbook

• ½ cup of pasta: the size of an ice cream scoop

• 1 cup of mashed potatoes: the size of your fist

• ½ bagel: the size of a hockey puck

• 1 ounce of cheese: the size of four stacked dice

• 1 medium fruit: the size of a tennis ball

• 1 ounce of pretzels or other snack foods: a large handful

• ½ cup of ice cream: the size of a tennis ball

food for fewer calories. By contrast, jelly beans—as well as croissants, chips, and doughnuts—have a high energy density and therefore a higher number of calories for their weight.

The lower a food's energy density, the fuller and more satisfied you'll feel, so you'll be less tempted to have seconds or thirds, says Barbara Rolls, Ph.D., professor of nutrition at Pennsylvania State University and author of *Volumetrics: Feel Full on Fewer Calories.*

Fruits, vegetables, and grains get their satisfying bulk from lots of water and fiber; they fill you up without filling you out, says Dr. Rolls.

They also tend to be high in complex carbohydrates, which increase blood sugar levels and signal the carbohydrate receptors in your body to tell your brain and belly that you've had enough food, thanks.

Here are a few ways nutritionists say you can modify recipes so they include less "dense" ingredients.

• If you make homemade pizza, avoid meat toppings, pile on the veggies, and reduce the amount of cheese.

• Add more beans and celery to chili and reduce the amount of ground beef.

• If you crave potato chips, dry-roasted peanuts, or corn chips, measure out 1 ounce—and eat with an apple.

4. Toss That Calculator

Here's a better idea than counting calories: Count *servings* of food, suggests Alphin. Your "calculator" is the government's Food Guide Pyramid, which calculates calories based on servings.

"If you follow the Food Guide Pyramid, you'll automatically eat sensible portions," says Alphin. You'll also maximize your intake of fiber,

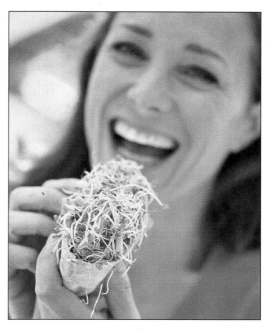

If you follow the **Food Guide** Pyramid, you'll automatically eat **sensible portions**.

essential vitamins and minerals, and the disease-fighting substances in plant foods.

Here's how Tartamella suggests you can translate healthy, weight-conscious eating guidelines into calories. If you're small and less active, opt for the lower-calorie allotments; if you're tall, big-boned, or active, pick the higher-calorie options. No matter which calorie amount you choose, limit your intake of fats, oils, and sweets.

To consume about 1,200 calories a day: Eat six servings of grains (at least three should be whole grains); three servings of vegetables; two servings of fruit; two servings of meat, poultry, fish, beans, eggs, or nuts; and two servings of milk, yogurt, or cheese (preferably low-fat).

To consume about 1,600 calories a day: Have eight servings of grain products (at least three should be whole grains); four servings of vegetables; three servings of fruit; two servings of meat, poultry, fish, beans, eggs, or nuts; and two servings of milk, yogurt, or cheese (preferably low-fat).

To consume about 2,000 calories a day: Eat nine servings of grains (at least three should be whole grains), five servings of vegetables, four servings of fruit, three servings of low-fat dairy products, and two 3-ounce portions of meat, poultry, or fish or two servings of beans, eggs, or nuts.

For calorie levels between the examples above, adjust the servings of grains, fruits, or vegetables, says Tartamella. Each serving of grains contains about 80 calories; fruit, about 60 calories; vegetables, about 25 calories. A serving of starchy vegetables (such as potatoes or corn) contains between 80 and 100 calories. So to move from 1,600 calories to 1,800 calories a day, you might have an extra piece of fruit at lunch, ½ cup of rice at dinner, and another piece of fruit as an evening snack.

Of course, counting servings trims calories only if you stick to the recommended serving sizes.

• *One serving of grains:* 1 slice of bread; ½ bagel or English muffin; 1 ounce cold cereal; ½ cup cooked cereal, rice, or pasta; 1 small roll, biscuit, or muffin; 2 large crackers.

1-MINUTE FAT BURNER

Pop a piece of gum. Researchers have recently discovered that chewing sugar-free gum all day increases your metabolic rate by about 20 percent. That could burn off more than 10 pounds a year.

• *One serving of fruit:* 1 medium apple, orange, or banana; ½ cup berries; ½ grapefruit; 1 slice of melon; ½ cup canned, chopped, or cooked fruit; ¾ cup fruit juice.

• *One serving of vegetables:* 1 cup raw leafy greens, ½ cup cooked vegetables, or ¾ cup vegetable juice.

• *One serving of dairy:* 1 cup milk or yogurt, 2 ounces processed cheese, 1½ ounces cheese.

• *One serving of meat, poultry, or fish:* 2 to 3 ounces. Count ½ cup cooked beans, 1 egg, 2 tablespoons nuts or peanut butter, or 4 ounces tofu as 1 serving of meat.

5. Burn, Ladies, Burn

Trimming calories is the "heads" side of the calorie equation. The "tails" side: *burning* calories. That's best accomplished by shedding fat and building muscle—in other words, exercise.

Exercise raises your resting metabolism by replacing do-nothing fat with calorie-burning muscle, explains Deborah Ezell, clinical exercise physiologist at the Johns Hopkins Weight Management Center in Baltimore. The more muscle you build, the more calories you'll burn, even while you sleep.

And even as you age.

Once we hit 40, we start replacing muscle with fat. In fact, we can expect to lose ½ pound of muscle every year during perimenopause and about 1 pound a year during menopause. This means that by the time you're 55, you could be down 15 pounds of muscle and burn about 600 fewer calories per day.

Scary thought. But exercise can help you turn back your metabolic clock—even after menopause.

Researchers at the University of Colorado in Boulder studied the metabolic rate of 65 pre-menopausal and postmenopausal women; 27 of them were sedentary, the rest were long-distance runners and swimmers. They found that, after menopause, the resting metabolism of the sedentary women dropped by about 130 calories a day. But the women who exercised had no drop in metabolic rate.

Muscle Up Your Metabolism

For pure calorie-burning power, you can't beat aerobic exercise, such as jogging, cycling, or cardio kickboxing.

"Aerobic exercise burns a lot of calories," says Ezell. "And when combined with eating fewer calories, it also promotes weight loss."

Further, aerobic exercise boosts your resting metabolism for several hours afterward, as your muscles burn calories to recover and repair themselves.

Say you're 150 pounds and you do vigorous aerobics for an hour. Besides the 558 calories you burn in that 60 minutes, you'll burn almost 100 more calories in the several hours following your workout, even if you're sprawled in front of the tube.

According to the American College of Sports Medicine, we should burn about 1,000 calories a week in physical activity. If you're 150

pounds, that translates to an hour of brisk walking three times a week.

Consider adding resistance training to your exercise program, too, says Ezell. "While resistance training doesn't burn many calories, it does build muscle," she says. "If you stick with it for over a year, you may eventually burn from 150 to 200 more calories a day." Her recommendation: Pump iron at least twice a week.

Aerobic exercise burns a lot of calories, and when combined with eating **fewer calories**, it also promotes weight loss.

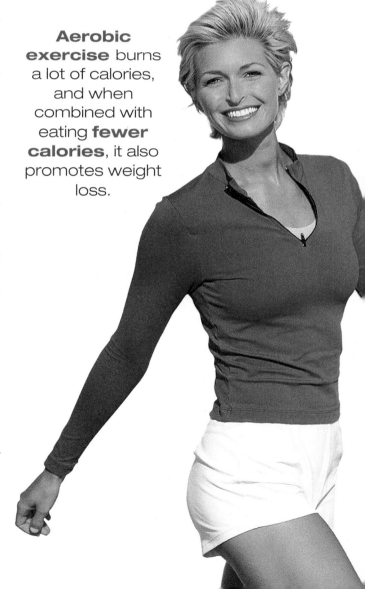

50 Ways to Shave 100 Calories

Eat just 100 extra calories a day—that's two chocolate sandwich cookies—and you'll be up 10 pounds in a year. But you can satisfy that cookie craving if you cut 100 calories from someplace else. Here are 50 painless ways to do it.

1. Instead of 1 cup of low-fat granola with raisins, have 1 cup of raisin bran.
2. Have a large caffe latte with fat-free milk instead of whole milk.
3. Have half a 4-ounce bagel with an orange, rather than the whole bagel.
4. Put 1 tablespoon of mustard on your turkey sandwich instead of 1¼ tablespoons of mayo.
5. Instead of 2 slices of cheese pizza, have veggie pizza (no cheese).
6. Order 2 slices of cheese pizza instead of 2 slices of pepperoni pizza.
7. Top your tossed salad with 3 tablespoons of fat-free ranch dressing instead of 2 tablespoons of full-fat dressing.
8. Try a veggie burger instead of a regular hamburger.
9. Have a cup of steamed rather than fried rice with your Chinese vegetables.
10. Put 1 less tablespoon of butter on your baked potato or use a margarine that's free of trans fats instead.
11. Instead of having 1 cup of macaroni and cheese and ½ cup of broccoli, reverse the amounts.
12. Eat only half of that slice of chocolate fudge cake with icing.
13. Instead of 6 cups of theater-style microwave popcorn, have the same amount of low-fat, butter-flavored microwave popcorn.
14. Spread 1 tablespoon of all-fruit jam on your toast rather than 1½ tablespoons of butter.
15. Instead of whole milk and eggs to prepare 2 slices of French toast, use fat-free milk and egg whites.
16. Munch on 1 ounce of baked minipretzels instead of 1 ounce of pecans.
17. Snack on an orange and a banana instead of a candy bar.
18. Steam asparagus rather than sautéing it in 1 tablespoon of butter or oil.
19. Replace 3 bacon slices with 3 slices of Light & Lean Canadian bacon.
20. Have 1 cup of vegetarian baked beans instead of 1 cup of baked beans with franks.
21. In sandwich spreads or salads, use 3 teaspoons of Dijonnaise instead of 4 teaspoons of mayonnaise.
22. Eat ½ cup of steamed fresh broccoli instead of ½ cup of frozen broccoli in cheese sauce.
23. Replace 1 cup of caramel-coated popcorn with 2½ cups of air-popped popcorn.

24. Stuff celery sticks with 2 tablespoons of fat-free cream cheese instead of 3 tablespoons of regular cream cheese.
25. Have 2 chocolate-chip cookies instead of 5.
26. Replace a 12-ounce can of cola with a 12-ounce can of diet cola.
27. Thicken your cream sauce with 1% milk and cornstarch instead of a roux of butter and flour.
28. Have 3 ounces of steak instead of 4½ ounces.
29. Grill a cheese sandwich with nonstick cooking spray instead of margarine.
30. Replace 1 cup of chocolate ice cream with ⅔ cup nonfat chocolate frozen yogurt.
31. Snack on 2 ounces of oven-baked potato chips instead of regular potato chips.
32. Instead of 1 cup macaroni salad, eat 3½ cups spinach salad with 2 tablespoons of low-calorie dressing.
33. Have 1 tablespoon of peanut butter on your sandwich instead of two.
34. Order a sandwich on cracked wheat bread instead of a croissant.
35. Snack on ½ cup of fruit cocktail canned in water instead of 1 cup of fruit cocktail canned in heavy syrup.
36. Dip your chips in ½ cup of salsa instead of ¾ cup of jalapeno cheese dip.
37. Use 1 tablespoon of mayonnaise instead of 3 tablespoons in your tuna salad.
38. Use 2 tablespoons of light pancake syrup instead of 2 tablespoons of regular syrup.
39. Top your pasta with 1 cup of marinara sauce instead of ¾ cup of Alfredo sauce.
40. Stop tasting as you cook. The following "tastes" have 100 calories: 4 tablespoons of beef Stroganoff, 3 tablespoons of homemade chocolate pudding, 2 tablespoons of chocolate-chip cookie dough.
41. Eat ¾ cup of pudding made with fat-free milk rather than 1 cup of pudding made with whole milk.
42. Snack on a papaya instead of a bag of M&M's.
43. Munch on 1 cup of frozen grapes instead of an ice cream sandwich.
44. When you have spaghetti, eat 2 meatballs instead of 4.
45. Choose 1 serving of vegetarian lasagna instead of lasagna with meat.
46. Eat 2 fruit and grain bars instead of 2 breakfast pastries.
47. Replace 1 large flour tortilla with a 6-inch corn tortilla.
48. Eat 1 hot dog, not 2, at a baseball game.
49. Order your hamburger without cheese.
50. Shred 2 ounces of fat-free Cheddar cheese on nachos instead of regular Cheddar.

More Sneaky Metabolism Boosters

There's no doubt that physical activity is the best way to rev up your body's metabolism. But it's not the only way. The following tips can help you crank your calorie-burning power to the max.

Don't crash. Those "drop a dress size in a week!" diets that are advertised in television commercials can slow metabolism by as much as 15 percent within the first 2 weeks, cautions Tartamella. So no matter how badly you want to lose weight, don't embark on any diet that offers fewer than 1,200 calories a day. "Drastically cutting calories makes your body think it's starving," explains Tartamella. "So it tries to conserve its energy stores by lowering the rate at which it burns calories."

Break your fast. You may be planning to eat lunch. But all your body knows is that it's not getting food—and may not for a long, long time. In order to conserve fuel, it starts burning calories more slowly. Eating breakfast reassures your body that there is no impending famine and that it's okay to "spend" its calories. In addition, eating breakfast helps keep you from overeating at lunch or dinner, according to Tartamella.

Eat often. Eat five or six mini-meals a day, or three squares plus two or three snacks of 100 to 200 calories each, recommends Tartamella. "Grazing" can also act as a binge-proofer, since eating lightly every few hours staves off hunger pangs.

Even if you consume the same number of calories, you'll burn them off better if you spread them throughout the day. Researchers at Tufts University in Boston found that older women

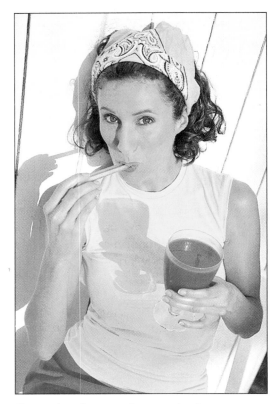

Drastically cutting calories **makes your body think it's starving**. So it tries to conserve its energy stores by lowering the rate at which it burns calories.

(their average age was 72) who ate mini-meals of 250 and 500 calories burned the same amount of calories as 25-year-old women. But when they consumed 1,000-calorie meals, they burned 60 fewer calories than the younger women. In just a year, that could add up to 6 pounds.

Let your period work for you. Two weeks before you begin to menstruate, your temperature rises, temporarily elevating your resting metabolism. During this time, you burn an average of 150 extra calories a day, and sometimes as many as 360 additional calories. So if you can withstand the premenstrual cravings, you will actually burn your own stored fat for energy.

Of course, don't compound PMS misery by denying yourself chocolate or chips, says Tartamella. "Better to have a small portion now than to binge later."

Muscle up your walks. Pumping your arms to chin height while you walk burns from 7 to 10 percent more calories than just walking regularly, according to John Porcari, Ph.D., professor in the department of exercise and sports science at the University of Wisconsin in La Crosse. "When you get your arms into the act, you're using more calorie-burning muscle."

Chapter 3

No More Excuses

25 solutions to 6 of the most common weight-loss dilemmas.

When it comes to weight loss, we can whip out a page of excuses longer than our weekend to-do list.

Often, what we think of as excuses are really solvable obstacles, says Karen Miller-Kovach, R.D., a registered dietitian and chief scientist for Weight Watchers International in Woodbury, New York. "Excuses are artificial," she says. "As soon as one is removed, another and another and another take its place. But obstacles have solutions that can resolve the problem. The key is finding the solution that is acceptable to you. Otherwise, you won't keep at it for the long term."

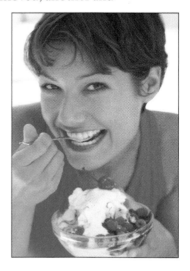

With that in mind, here are some excuse-busters: solid, simple-to-follow solutions for overcoming the most common weight-loss obstacles. Learn how to stop cravings before they start, make exercise automatic, get the body you want, eat your favorite foods without gaining weight, and triumph over temptations.

1. "I'm dying for a hot fudge sundae."

Cutting way back on calories, skipping meals, or vowing to never again eat chocolate may help you drop pounds fast, but it will ultimately undo your success. "Quick-fix, short-term thinking can trip you up," says Diane Grabowski-Nepa, R.D., a registered dietitian and nutrition educator at the Pritikin Longevity Center in Santa Monica, California.

The more you deprive yourself, the stronger—and harder to resist—your cravings become. The same is true if you're eating the same thing day after day, no matter how healthy it is.

"If you're bored with your food, you're

11 Warning Signs That You're About to Falter

Check off the scenarios below to see if you might be close to falling off the wagon. Score one point for each check mark and then add up your score.

☐ 1. You've stopped writing in your food journal.

☐ 2. You feel hopeless about your weight after treating yourself to cookies 3 days in a row.

☐ 3. You feel deprived and sorry for yourself because your plan is so restrictive.

☐ 4. You've eaten broiled chicken and steamed veggies 5 nights this week.

☐ 5. You feel guilty when you eat anything except fruits and veggies.

☐ 6. You skip exercise when you're busy, instead of squeezing in a 15-minute workout.

☐ 7. You suddenly feel the urge to nap—at your usual workout time.

☐ 8. You "forget" to put your gym bag in the car.

☐ 9. You tell yourself that walking to and from the mailbox is enough exercise for the day.

☐ 10. You skip the gym to work late—even when you don't have an urgent deadline or big project.

☐ 11. You pull into the nearly full health club parking lot, conclude that all of the treadmills are taken, and pull right out again.

TOTAL _____

Here's how to interpret your score. If you scored zero to 2, great job! Keep up the good work! A score of 3 to 5 calls for caution. You're hitting a dip in your motivation level. A score of 6 or more means you're on dangerous ground. Keep this book with you at all times.

eating the wrong food," says Nancy Clark, R.D., of Brookline, Massachusetts, a registered dietitian and author of *Nancy Clark's Sports Nutrition Guidebook*. You won't stick with any diet if you don't like the food. Here's how to enjoy healthy eating and stop those cravings.

Don't give up on your favorites. With careful planning, you can have chocolate, ice cream, or any other high-calorie, high-fat treat and still lose weight. "The key is to eat what you want, and mind the portions," says Ronette L. Kolotkin, Ph.D., clinical psychologist at the Duke University Diet and Fitness Center in Durham, North Carolina. She recalls a client who lost—and kept off—100 pounds, even though he never gave up his love of pizza. "He knew from past dieting experiences that giving it up completely wouldn't last, so he found a way to fit it into his long-term plan."

Fuel your body. Think of your diet strategy as fueling your body. Eating frequently in small amounts throughout the day and evening helps avoid the hunger that leads to temptation.

Expand your culinary skills. Learning how to prepare food will help you appreciate it more, and make it easier for you to stick with a pleasurable eating plan. Take a class on low-fat cooking, or ask a friend who has lost weight to share her recipes and ideas.

Be adventurous. Buy at least one new healthy food—an exotic grain such as quinoa for pilaf instead of rice, or interesting produce such

> # 1-MINUTE FAT BURNER
>
> **Post inspiration. To keep yourself on track, place quotes in strategic spots where you might need some motivation: on the fridge, TV, dashboard, or computer. A suggestion: "You've come too far to take orders from a cookie."**

as jicama or star fruit—every time you go shopping. If you like it, incorporate it into your usual meal plans. If not, try something else next time.

Make it easy. Invest in low-fat cooking tools—nonstick pots and pans, a rice cooker, a vegetable steamer, and a garlic press. These kitchen gadgets make healthy-meal preparation easier and more enjoyable.

2. "I'm not seeing results."

You're doing everything right. So why has your progress stalled? In a *Prevention*/NBC *Today* survey, 70 percent of the women polled reported hitting a weight-loss plateau, despite following their diet and exercise programs to the letter.

"A plateau is your body's way of acclimating to a new weight in a healthy way," Grabowski-Nepa says. Think of it as the weight-loss equivalent of a climber who is ascending Mt. Everest resting at different levels for a few days until her body gets used to the altitude. If you've been in a holding pattern for more than 2 weeks, however, here's how to take yourself to the next level.

Mix things up. Learn to play tennis or any other activity that you've never tried before. Doing the same type of exercise day after day, week after week, can actually decrease the number of calories you burn. Your muscles become more efficient, so they don't have to work as hard. Variety will keep muscles at their calorie-burning max.

Keep a diary. Now is a good time to revisit your exercise and eating habits. Once the pounds start coming off, it's easy to slip back into old habits: having dessert more often, shortening your walks, or skipping them altogether. Keeping a food and activity log may be all you need to get back on track.

Throw away the scale. Instead, focus on the increased energy you now have, how easy it is to race up a flight of stairs, the way your favorite skirt no longer digs into your tummy, or the decrease in your blood pressure. The scale is not your best measure of success. In fact, if you're strength training (which we highly recommend), the scale may actually go up a bit because you're building muscle. Don't panic! While muscle may weigh a bit more than fat, it looks a lot better and burns calories like crazy!

Get a new weight-loss plan. What helped you to lose the first 10, 30, or even 50 pounds may not be the right way to lose your last 10, 30, or even 50 pounds. So you may need to make some adjustments, such as exercising a bit more or eating a little differently. Including more fruit, salads, vegetables, and vegetable-based soups at lunch, dinner, and snack time can help you fill up on fewer calories while dropping pounds.

Rethink your goal. Before you get worked up about those last 5 or 10 pounds, ask

If you hate what you're doing and can't wait to stop, **that's not the right kind of exercise** for you.

yourself whether you may already be at your ideal weight. You may not achieve your goal *weight*. But if you look and feel great, you certainly have achieved your goal.

3. "I can't stick with exercise."

Going from a couch potato—or even an occasional exerciser—to walking, jogging, or cycling

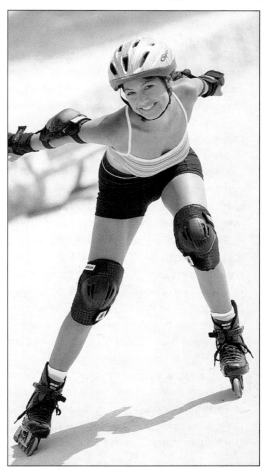

Weight Loss
HELP OR HYPE?

An Answer to Cellulite

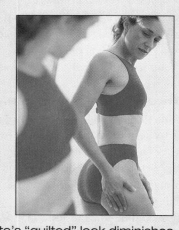

Can you really just massage away cellulite? The FDA gave the okay for the makers of Endermologie, a deep-suctioning massage device first approved in 1996, to claim it's an "effective treatment for temporarily reducing the appearance of cellulite." Considering the other cellulite products that were rejected in the past, we wanted to know more.

According to its manufacturer, Endermologie works by stretching and relaxing connective fibers that link fat and skin. As blood circulation increases and water buildup is eliminated, the cellulite's "quilted" look diminishes.

There's one important detail: You're instructed to eat low-fat foods, drink ten 8-ounce glasses of water a day, and exercise.

"It's hard to know how much of the results are due simply to the diet and exercise," says Deborah Sarnoff, M.D., assistant clinical professor in the department of dermatology at New York University Medical Center in New York City, who has conducted informal Endermologie studies at her Manhattan private practice and seen "very nice results."

Researchers studied this procedure at Vanderbilt University's School of Medicine in Nashville. There, Yucatan mini pigs, chosen for their skin's likeness to that of humans, underwent up to 20 Endermologie sessions on one side of their bodies. Skin biopsies revealed "what appeared to be new collagen deposited horizontally in the deepest layer of skin tissue," which could be why some people see positive results, says David Adcock, M.D., a researcher on the study. But there's no guarantee yet that human skin will react in the same way.

While Endermologie probably can't do much physical damage (you could be bruised if the technician accidentally applies too much pressure), it might make your wallet wince. At roughly $1,400—about $100 for each session, with at least 14 sessions needed—it's a hefty outlay for a procedure that promises only a temporary improvement. "But if nothing else, it's an invigorating, wonderful massage," says Dr. Sarnoff.

almost daily is a big commitment. But you can do it if you avoid some common traps. A sure-fire way to end up back on the couch is to choose an activity that rates on the excitement meter with folding laundry. If you don't enjoy it, you won't commit. Another is doing too much, too fast. Trying to keep up with your husband who runs 5-Ks or going for a 25-mile bike ride could leave you feeling bad about yourself—or with sore muscles or an injury. Here's how to love exercise and make it as regular as brushing your teeth.

Learn to crawl. If your primary form of exercise has been doing laps around the grocery aisles once a week, it's unrealistic to expect yourself to power walk for an hour a day. But it's not impossible—with time. Break your goal down into smaller, more manageable bits. "I know one woman who started exercising for 5 minutes at a time," says Dr. Kolotkin. "By feeling positive about it and patting herself on the back, she gradually worked her way up to walking marathons."

Play around. Look at your first workouts as experiments, not commitments, suggests Dr. Kolotkin. (You're committed to exercising, but not in any particular form.) "If you hate what you're doing and you can't wait to stop, that's not the right kind of exercise for you," she says. Pick three activities that interest you—maybe kickboxing, inline skating, and swimming. Then try each one, individually, for at least a week. Chances are that you'll like one and can have fun mastering it. If not, try some others.

Forget the sweat. If you hate the thought of exercise because you envision a huffing, puffing, shirt-drenching workout, go the moderate route. You can burn loads of calories with activities that are less strenuous. Try walking, dancing, golf, or gardening.

Celebrate! Changing habits is hard work, so reward yourself along the way. Didn't miss a single walk last week? Treat yourself to those cute sandals you've been eyeing. Made it all the way through an hour-long step class? Buy yourself a big bouquet of flowers. Began a strength-training program? Schedule a massage. Choose anything that feels like a reward.

Double your pleasure. If you cherish a good book, want to spend more time with your kids, or meet friends regularly, make these part of your workout. Sign up for an exercise class with a friend. Take the kids hiking. Listen to books on tape while you use the treadmill. The added incentive will help to make you a regular exerciser.

4. "I might as well eat the whole box now."

"Psychologists call this the 'what-the-hell' effect," says Andrea Dunn, Ph.D., an exercise psychologist at the Cooper Institute for Aerobics Research in Dallas. "It happens when you've started to change a poor habit, but then make a mistake. You have a fast-food burger and then think, 'What the hell, I've already blown it. I might as well eat the fries, too.'"

The same phenomenon occurs with exercise. You miss a workout or two, decide the whole thing is a loss, and never go back to the gym. But the idea that you've blown anything is false, Dr. Dunn says. "You haven't failed if you eat something high calorie or miss a workout; you've just had a momentary lapse." Here's how to keep a brief tumble off the weight-loss wagon from turning into a colossal failure.

Save your pennies. Every time you do something right, put a penny in a big glass jar. Passed on the doughnuts at work? Add a penny. Walked 30 minutes on the treadmill? Another penny. Ate three pieces of fruit today? Another. Then, when you have a slipup, put a penny in a different jar. Over time, you'll see that most of the time you're doing well. It's the big picture that counts.

Don't overreact. After bingeing at your neighbor's Fourth of July picnic, the worst thing you could do is starve yourself the next day. Yes, in theory it seems that doing so might compensate for all of the calories you ate yesterday, but you're actually setting yourself up for another binge. The best strategy: Get back to your normal eating and exercise plan as soon as possible.

Give yourself a pep talk. A big part of changing behaviors is changing the way we think. Instead of berating yourself for eating a brownie or missing a workout, be positive. Tell yourself, "I'm doing well. I'm really making progress." Say it out loud for more emphasis!

Playing the Numbers Game

When picking a goal weight, people tend to make two mistakes. They either pick a weight they have to torture themselves to get to, or they have a lot of weight to lose, so they pick a daunting, long-term weight-loss goal, such as 50 pounds or more, says Ross Andersen, Ph.D., of the Johns Hopkins University Weight Management Center in Baltimore.

In the first case, Dr. Andersen says, even those who make it to their target weights find that they can't stay there. "It's one thing to diet down to a certain weight. Some people can't keep it there, but they still think that is their ideal weight," Dr. Andersen says.

In the second case, setting a goal that seems so far away can overwhelm people before they even begin. "That's part of a big problem. They say, 'I've got so much to lose, I don't know how to get started,'" Dr. Andersen says.

That's why Dr. Andersen has developed a strategy for choosing a weight-loss goal. It takes into account both common mistakes. It allows you to lose a reasonable amount of weight that you'll be able to maintain. Also, it breaks a major weight-loss goal down into smaller pieces, making it seem much less daunting. Here's how to choose a weight-loss goal that you can reach and maintain.

Go to the 5 and 10. A weight-loss goal of 5 to 10 percent of your total weight is considered a huge success. Even if you want to lose much more, start

5. "My husband keeps bringing home ice cream."

Unsupportive family, friends, and coworkers can make weight loss even tougher, says Susan J. Bartlett, Ph.D., a clinical psychologist who treats weight disorders at the Johns Hopkins School of Medicine in Baltimore. "But that type of frontal assault is the exception, not the rule," she says. More often, you'll face a more subtle sabotage: the sniping from people who resent your success and are looking for ways to register their jealousy or hurt feelings. This sometimes happens if your new schedule means you have less time to spend with them. Here's how to get the support you need.

Start talking. You need to be frank about what you see happening and how it's affecting you. Many times the other person isn't even aware that she's sabotaging your efforts and doesn't understand that you need her support, says Dr. Bartlett. "Often, those who've never had to lose weight have no concept of how hard it is."

Compromise. If you're spending less time with friends because you've sworn off girls'

with this goal, Dr. Andersen says. With this percentage, you'll see health and appearance differences, but it isn't so drastic a goal that it is unattainable or unmanageable. So if you are 160 pounds, your initial weight-loss goal will be 8 to 16 pounds.

Strive for 1 to 2 pounds a week on average. Make the lifestyle changes recommended in this book, and you'll shed 1 to 2 pounds a week. Rapid weight loss is usually done through drastic measures, so that once you go back to life as you knew it, the weight returns as quickly as you lost it. A slow, steady weight loss is not only healthier but also easier to keep off, Dr. Andersen says.

Just keep this in mind, he advises: Think about your weight loss on average over the course of time, instead of worrying about how many pounds you lost in one particular week. One week, you may lose only 1 pound, but the next week, you may lose 3 pounds.

Keep it off for a while. Once you reach your 5-to-10-percent goal, your next goal should be maintaining your new weight, Dr. Andersen says. For many, keeping the weight off is the real challenge. By spending a few weeks or months simply staying at your new weight, you give your body and yourself a breather from the mental and physical rigors of trying to lose weight.

This maintenance period also allows you to make sure that lifestyle changes become just that: permanent changes that you'll carry with you the rest of your life, not just changes you made for short-term weight loss.

night out at the coffeehouse with the double fudge cheesecake you just can't resist, suggest meeting someplace with fewer temptations. Or better yet, do something active together: a stroll through the park or a night out dancing.

Don't sermonize. Nothing is more annoying than a fresh convert, so spare your friends and family the diatribe about how healthy you've become. "When you preach, you're putting yourself up on a holier-than-thou pedestal," says Grabowski-Nepa. "And people will only knock you down." Yes, you should be proud of yourself. Just don't try to constantly convert others.

6. "I just don't have time."

After a busy day of pleasing the boss, keeping the house running smoothly, and chauffeuring the kids, a trip through the drive-thru and an evening on the couch may sound appealing. But it won't do anything to get you back into that little black dress you love.

Marathon runners don't have more time than you, but they manage to cram in workouts. They do something that you can, too: Make exercise a priority, a nonnegotiable part of your life. Here's how.

Pen it in. Take a look at your day planner and decide where you have some extra time—even 10 minutes is a start. If every day is crammed, decide what can go. Be ruthless: Do you really need to socialize at every lunch hour? Or sleep in as late as possible every day?

Buy convenience foods. Stock up on frozen, low-cal dinners and low-fat canned soups—and then hit the rest of the store for precut vegetables, salads in a bag, and low-fat dressings and sauces to spoon over a baked potato or chicken breast. "This stuff is as easy as fast food," says Grabowski-Nepa. "All you need is a microwave and a spoon."

Get moving—early. Schedule your workouts for the first thing in the morning. "We know that people who exercise earlier in the day are more likely to be regular exercisers," says Dr. Bartlett. "We suspect that's because the later in the day you schedule it, the more likely it is that things will come up to prevent you from doing it."

Do two things at once. "Patients tell me that they look for opportunities to combine physical activity with other necessary evils. For instance, many now have 'active meetings' at work: Instead of sitting around a conference table, they take a walk while addressing routine office issues," says Dr. Bartlett.

Changing habits is hard work, so **reward yourself along the way.** Choose anything that feels like a reward.

LIFESTYLE RESTYLE

She Ate to Relieve Stress

Carole DeMartino, a 55-year-old laboratory manager from Bloomfield, New Jersey, calls her 120-pound weight loss a midlife miracle. Dieting, she says, has nothing to do with your stomach and everything to do with your brain.

DeMartino got fat when she was 2 years old, and stayed fat. "When I was a child, I used to go to sleep praying for a miracle—that I'd wake up and the rest of the world would be fat, too," she says.

She went on her first diet when she was in eighth grade. Her mother took her to the doctor, and he prescribed amphetamines. "Of course I lost weight; I didn't eat or sleep. But as soon as I went off the pills, the weight came back. By the time I got to high school, my nickname was Carole Barrel," she remembers.

Growing up fat was stressful, and she learned to use food to soothe that stress. On the outside, DeMartino was a jolly, flamboyant fat person. But she was miserable on the inside, she says. No one saw her eat. She'd skip meals all day, and then go home and pig out every night.

"Food was my comfort. I became a food addict. One spoonful of ice cream was too much and a half-gallon wasn't enough. My life was one big eating marathon," she says.

One day, she decided it was time to step on the scale. DeMartino's weight—265 pounds—shocked her into the recognition that she was killing herself. "Because I manage a medical lab, I knew all along that my numbers weren't good. I was 50 years old and had high blood pressure, high blood sugar, and extremely high cholesterol. I realized at that point something had to be done," she recalls.

She started out by saying, "Let's see what I can do one day at a time." She went on a cabbage soup diet and lost 15 pounds. That was all she needed to get started. After that, DeMartino adopted a low-fat, high-carbohydrate eating plan and eventually became a vegetarian. In 18 months, she lost 120 pounds.

Instead of eating to cope with stress, she exercised everyday, starting out with simply walking around the block. Now, DeMartino lifts weights twice a week and walks for an hour each day. "I've never felt better. My blood pressure and blood sugar are normal and my cholesterol is down to 180," she says.

"Being thin hasn't made stress evaporate from my life, but I've learned to deal with it differently. Some nights, I come home from work so stressed that I'm just crying to eat. I've found a way to break that cycle. I rinse my mouth out with water or brush my teeth. Then I go for a 60-minute walk. All of that negative energy dissipates and is replaced by positive energy. Exercise is just plain good for your soul."

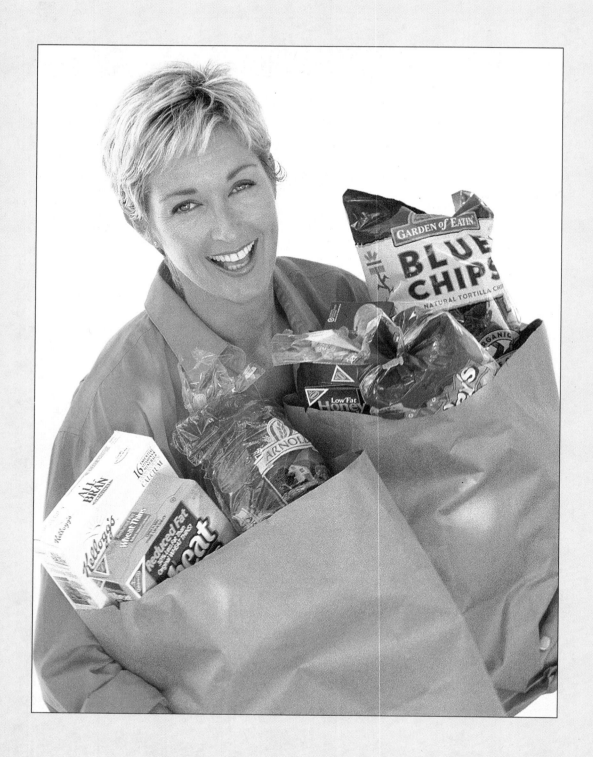

Part Two

Eat Right
for Life

Chapter 4

Discover the Power of Positive Eating

Inspired to eat right? We'll show you how in 10 easy steps.

What better time than right now to give your body a new lease on life? Our Positive-Eating Plan has all you need to make a fresh start toward fabulous health. This exclusive plan combines the best of the best: It brings you every top nutrition strategy likely to increase your chances of reaping the joys of good health and achieving slow, steady weight loss (the type that lasts).

This is not a good diet—it's the ultimate diet.

Is it easy? Quite honestly, because this eating plan represents the ultimate in nutrition, you'll probably find it a challenge at first, as you adopt some new, powerfully healthy habits. But the results will be worth it. Studies show that choosing the foods in this diet should lower your risk of heart attack, high blood pressure, stroke, cancer, diabetes, osteoporosis, cataracts, obesity, asthma, diverticulosis, depression, and even PMS. You may even achieve a longer, better life.

The Basics of the Plan

Quite simply, the Positive-Eating Plan emphasizes the foods that are good for you rather than worrying about the ones that aren't. It's designed to deliver 1,500 calories a day, a level that will result in gradual weight loss for most women. On the plan, you'll eat six mini-meals a day of about 250 calories each. Not only does this eating style prevent dips in energy but it also appears to help you burn calories better as you grow older. For women over 50, this could prevent a weight gain of up to 6 pounds a year.

If you need more than 1,500 calories a day, double the portions for one or more mini-meals.

Read on to learn the 10 steps to positive eating, and start following them today.

1: Eat Nine Servings of Vegetables and Fruits Every Day

Veggies and fruits are the foundation of the Positive-Eating Plan, as opposed to grains, the foundation of the traditional Food Pyramid. You'll be eating nine ½-cup servings of a variety of fruits and veggies each day.

Does that sound like overkill? In reality, it could mean extra life. Study after study links the diets that are highest in fruits and vegetables with fewer cancers and less heart disease, diabetes, and even osteoporosis. The landmark DASH (Dietary Approaches

Five Tips That Make Mini-Meals Work

1. **Keep the *mini* in *mini-meals*.** Buy snack foods in single serving sizes so you won't be tempted to overeat. Divvy up big bags of crackers into snack-size plastic bags.
2. **Stock mini-meals at work.** Here are some desk-drawer ideas: packets of instant oatmeal, instant soup cups, and whole-grain crackers. Or stash low-fat yogurt, baby carrots, and tomato juice in the lunchroom fridge.
3. **Travel with mini-meals.** Stash nonperishable goodies such as small boxes of raisins, cans of vegetable juice cocktail, and whole-wheat pretzels in your car, purse, or briefcase.
4. **Turn the evening meal into "family dessert."** If everyone comes home hungry at different times, can older teens and parents fix and eat healthy mini-meal dinners on their own. Gather later to eat your mini-meal dessert or evening snack together as a family.
5. **Find mini-meals on menus.** If there's an appetizer that appeals to you, have it as a mini-meal. Many restaurants let you order an appetizer instead of an entrée. If not, eat half of your entrée (or less, if it's huge), and take the rest home.

to Stop Hypertension) diet study found that nine servings a day lowered blood pressure as much as some prescription drugs.

More and more experts are saying that five servings a day should be the minimum and that nine a day—five vegetables and four fruits—is the optimum. Yet most Americans get only four a day. On the Positive-Eating Plan, you'll need to make every meal and snack a fruit or veggie opportunity.

Quick tip: Use time-saving frozen and canned veggies and fruits, which provide the same nutrients as fresh produce.

2. Eat Three to Six Whole Grain Foods Every Day

Diets high in whole grains are linked to less heart disease and diabetes and fewer strokes and cancers. If you've been eating a high-carbohydrate diet with lots of refined grains, typically breads, rolls, bagels, pretzels, and crackers made from white flour, it may be a challenge at first to find whole grain substitutes.

But the payoff is worth it. To your body, refined white flour is the same as sugar, making a diet high in white flour foods the same as a high-sugar diet. Start reading the ingredient lists of all of your grain products. Choose the ones made with a whole grain; you should see the actual word *whole*.

Quick tip: To find whole wheat bread, check the ingredients list; the first ingredient should be whole wheat flour.

1-MINUTE FAT BURNER

Mix a juice spritzer. Combine your favorite juice (half your usual amount) with plain or sparkling water. You can cut up to 85 calories per glass—and lose 5 pounds or more a year.

---

3. Eat Two or Three Calcium-Rich Foods Every Day

Not only does adequate calcium support strong bones and help prevent osteoporosis, but clinical studies suggest that it helps prevent colon cancer, high blood pressure, and PMS.

Obvious high-calcium choices include 1% and fat-free milk, low-fat and fat-free yogurt, and reduced-fat and fat-free cheese. Other good choices are orange and grapefruit juices and soy milk that have been fortified with calcium. To equal the calcium found in milk, look for at least 30 percent of the Daily Value (DV) for calcium per serving.

Quick tip: If you are lactose intolerant, try dairy products that are lactose-free.

4. Eat Beans Five or More Times a Week

Beans are the highest-fiber foods you can find, with the single exception of breakfast cereals made with wheat bran. Diets high in fiber are linked to less cancer, heart disease, and diabetes, and fewer strokes and even ulcers. Beans are especially high in soluble fiber, which lowers cholesterol levels, and folate, which lowers levels of another risk factor for heart disease: homocysteine.

Quick tip: To reduce sodium in canned beans by about one-third, drain off the canning liquid and rinse them before using. Or look for canned beans with no added sodium.

Give Yourself a Quick Fiber Checkup

If the typical person doubled her fiber intake, she could lose 9 to 10 pounds over the course of a year without lowering her calorie intake. How? Fiber cuts calories by blocking the digestion of some of the fat and protein consumed with it.

Think of fiber as many fine threads. As they travel through the intestinal tract, the threads wrap around each other like a piece of twine, tying up calories in the process. For best results, aim for 30 grams of fiber daily, spread out over the day.

Fiber cuts calories in more straightforward ways as well. Most high-fiber foods are low in calories and fat, so if you eat more of them, you'll eat fewer calories and less fat. And because of their bulk, high-fiber foods tend to satisfy hunger quickly, before you have a chance to overeat.

Use this easy counter to see if you're getting 30 grams of fiber each day. Fill in the number of servings of each particular food you eat each day, multiply it by the number of grams of fiber, and then add up all your answers.

1.5 grams of fiber × _____ servings of fruit = _____ grams

1.5 grams of fiber × _____ servings of vegetables = _____ grams

2.5 grams of fiber × _____ servings of whole grains (whole wheat bread and pasta or brown rice) = _____ grams

1 gram of fiber × _____ servings of refined grains (white bread and pasta or white rice) = _____ grams

5 grams of fiber × _____ servings of dried beans = _____ grams

_____ grams of fiber in a serving of your breakfast cereal × _____ servings of cereal = _____ grams

Your total daily fiber intake = _____ grams

5. Eat Nuts Five Times a Week

Studies show that people who eat nuts regularly have less heart disease and fewer other illnesses than people who avoid them. Even among the healthiest eaters, the ones who also eat nuts have the best health records. Exactly why isn't known yet, but one reason could be compounds in nuts called tocotrienols.

The key to eating nuts is to not eat too many; they're so high in calories that you could easily gain weight. To avoid temptation, we suggest keeping a jar of chopped nuts in your fridge. Sprinkle 2 tablespoons a day on cereal, yogurt, veggies, salads, or wherever the crunch and rich flavor appeal to you.

Quick tip: Be sure to store nuts in the refrigerator to keep them from oxidizing and turning rancid.

6. Eat Fish Twice a Week

Studies show that people who eat fish twice a week are less likely to have fatal heart attacks. Scientists credit omega-3 fatty acids, which have the ability to prevent the development of a dangerously irregular heartbeat.

Humans evolved on diets that supplied more omega-3's than we get today, and some experts suspect that rising rates of depression have been caused by a lack of omega-3's in brain cell membranes.

To get the most omega-3's, choose salmon, white albacore tuna canned in water, rainbow trout, anchovies, herring, sardines, and mackerel.

Quick tip: You can get a plant version of omega-3 fat in canola oil.

7. Drink Eight Glasses of Water Every Day, Plus a Cup or More of Tea

Every cell in your body needs water to function. And big water drinkers appear to get fewer colon and bladder cancers. Drinking lots of water helps you feel full, too.

In addition, every cup of tea provides a strong infusion of antioxidants that help keep blood from clotting too easily (which may thwart heart attacks) and may help lower your risk of cancer and rheumatoid arthritis.

Quick tip: Both green and black tea contain powerful antioxidants.

8. Keep a Fat Budget

To stay within a healthy fat budget (25 percent of calories from fat), you must first find the maximum fat allowance for your calorie level.

Maximum Fat Allowance

Calories	Fat (g)
1,250	35
1,500	42
1,750	49
2,000	56

Once you know your fat budget, see whether you are staying within its bounds. Add up the grams of fat in all the food that you eat in a day. Almost all food labels will tell you the grams of total fat in a serving.

"The Positive-Eating Menus" on page 42 are designed to have approximately 42 grams of fat, the healthy limit for a 1,500-calorie diet.

Try to get most of your fat from olive and canola oils (or salad dressings made from them), nuts, fish, and margarine that's free of trans fats. And spread your fat throughout the day; a little fat helps you absorb fat-soluble nutrients from vegetables and fruits. To avoid trans fats, which raise cholesterol, read the ingredient lists of any processed foods that you buy. If you see the words *partially hydrogenated*, look for a different product.

9. Take Some Sensible Nutrition Insurance

Besides beginning your fabulous diet, take a multivitamin/mineral supplement, plus 100 to

400 IU of vitamin E and 100 to 500 milligrams of vitamin C. On days when you eat only two calcium-rich foods, take 500 milligrams of calcium if you're under age 50; take 1,000 milligrams of calcium (divided into two separate doses of 500 milligrams each) if you're 50 or older.

Key Supplements

Supplement	Daily Dosage
Multivitamin/mineral	100% DV for most nutrients
Calcium	Under 50 years old: 500 mg*
	Over 50 years old: 1,000 mg*
Vitamin E	100–400 IU
Vitamin C	100–500 mg

*You will need 500 milligrams more than these amounts if you're not eating high-calcium foods.

10. Consider Your Options Carefully

Decisions about eating the following foods are up to you with the Positive-Eating Plan.

Meat and poultry. You can eat up to 3 cooked ounces (the size of a deck of playing cards) per day. You will get enough protein on the plan without adding meat, and studies consistently link vegetarian diets to better health, perhaps partly because diets low in meat are naturally lower in saturated fat.

Eggs. If you have diabetes or high cholesterol or are overweight, you can eat up to four eggs a week; if you have none of these conditions, up to seven eggs a week is okay.

Alcohol. Experts condone the intake of up to one drink a day for women. (One drink is the equivalent of 5 ounces of wine, 12 ounces of

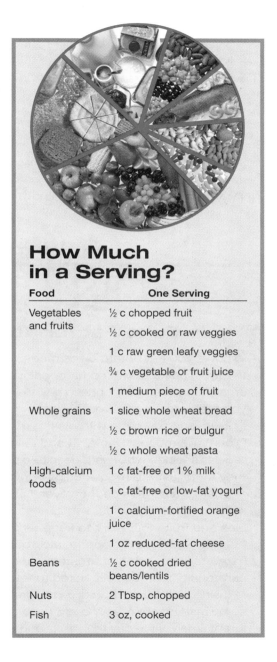

How Much in a Serving?

Food	One Serving
Vegetables and fruits	½ c chopped fruit
	½ c cooked or raw veggies
	1 c raw green leafy veggies
	¾ c vegetable or fruit juice
	1 medium piece of fruit
Whole grains	1 slice whole wheat bread
	½ c brown rice or bulgur
	½ c whole wheat pasta
High-calcium foods	1 c fat-free or 1% milk
	1 c fat-free or low-fat yogurt
	1 c calcium-fortified orange juice
	1 oz reduced-fat cheese
Beans	½ c cooked dried beans/lentils
Nuts	2 Tbsp, chopped
Fish	3 oz, cooked

beer, or 1½ ounces of 80-proof distilled spirits such as gin, rum, or vodka.) Studies show that moderate consumption of alcohol, especially red wine, lowers the risk of heart disease. But it also slightly raises the risk of breast cancer.

Sweets. Reserve these for special occasions. Positive eating means loading your every calorie with life-enhancing nutrition. High-sugar foods provide empty calories and little else. People who avoid all sugar for a month or two often find that they lose their cravings for it. It's worth trying.

The Positive-Eating Menus

Here are 3 days' worth of easy and delicious menus to help you get started on your Positive-Eating Plan.

Weight Loss
HELP OR HYPE?

Is Fake Fat for You?

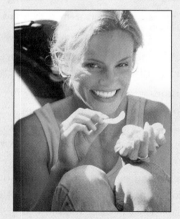

Should you eat potato chips made with olestra, the fat substitute with no fat or calories? Only in small quantities, only once in a while, and only if you really, really want to.

True, snacks made with olestra (brand name Olean) are much lower in fat and calories than regular snacks, which is a definite plus. And they taste just like regular chips—another plus.

There's a down side, however. Olestra siphons off carotenoids, substances in vegetables and fruits that work to keep us disease-free. For example, lycopene, a carotenoid in tomatoes and red grapefruit, is linked to lower rates of prostate cancer and heart disease. Lutein, a carotenoid in broccoli, is linked to fewer cataracts.

Inside you, olestra hooks on to carotenoids in your digestive tract and escorts some of them out of your body, unabsorbed. Even if you eat olestra chips at different times of the day than fruits and vegetables, your uptake of carotenoids could be reduced by as much as 10 percent. And you need more carotenoids, not fewer. Until we know more about olestra, it makes sense to go easy with it.

Day 1

Diet tip: Choosing fruits and vegetables with vivid colors helps you zero in on the nutrient powerhouses.

Breakfast: ½ of a grapefruit and one slice of whole-wheat toast with 1 tablespoon of fruit spread

Midmorning snack: ¾ of a cup of Concord grape juice, 1 cup of oatmeal, and 1 cup of fat-free milk

Lunch: 1 cup of black bean soup, one wedge of cornbread, and 1 cup of spinach salad topped with ½ cup of orange sections

Midafternoon snack: 1 ounce of reduced-fat Cheddar cheese, 2 tablespoons of walnuts, and an apple

Dinner: 1 cup of cooked whole wheat pasta shells with 1 tablespoon of olive oil, two cloves of garlic, 1 cup of broccoli, and ½ cup of red bell pepper slices

Evening snack: 1 cup of reduced-sodium tomato juice cocktail and four whole wheat crackers

Day's total: 1,506 calories, 45 grams of fat, 10 grams of saturated fat, 23 grams of fiber, and 2,168 milligrams of sodium

Day 2

Diet tip: No doubt about it, homemade shakes and smoothies are the most delicious way to get your fruit and calcium.

Breakfast: ¾ of a cup of hot whole wheat cereal; ½ cup of frozen blueberries, thawed; and 1 cup of fat-free milk

Midmorning snack: 1 slice of toasted raisin bread with 1 tablespoon of natural peanut butter

Lunch: 1 small bean burrito, and eight grape tomatoes halved and tossed with 2

Servings

Food	Servings
Daily	
Vegetables and fruits	9 (5 veggies/4 fruits)
Whole grains	3–6
High-calcium foods	2–3
Water	8 glasses
Tea	1 cup or more
Weekly	
Beans	5+
Nuts	5
Fish	2

ounces of crumbled reduced-fat feta cheese

Midafternoon snack: 1 serving of Papaya Power Shake (see page 45)

Dinner: 2 ounces of roast chicken breast, 1 cup of mashed butternut squash, 1 cup of brussels sprouts, and ½ cup of corn kernels mixed with ¼ cup of cooked barley and 2 teaspoons of canola oil

Evening snack: 1 extra-large baked apple with 2 teaspoons of honey or brown sugar

Day's total: 1,529 calories, 45 grams of fat, 15 grams of saturated fat, 30 grams of fiber, and 2,609 milligrams of sodium

Day 3

Diet tip: Make sure that you eat vegetables with a little fat, such as salad dressing or reduced-fat cheese. You'll absorb more nutrients.

Breakfast: ½ of a toasted whole wheat bagel topped with ¼ cup of reduced-fat ricotta cheese and three finely chopped prunes

Midmorning snack: 1 cup of low-fat plain yogurt with half of a banana, sliced, and 1 tablespoon of chopped walnuts

Lunch: Pasta salad made with 1 cup of

cooked whole wheat rotini or pasta spirals; ½ cup of broccoli; ½ cup of yellow bell pepper; half of a tomato, chopped; 1 tablespoon of olive oil, and 1 teaspoon of vinegar

Midafternoon snack: 2 rye crispbread sheets, 2 tablespoons of light cream cheese, and ½ cup of frozen strawberries, thawed

Dinner: 1 serving of Carrot Soup with Lime and Chiles (see below), six large shrimp broiled with 1 tablespoon of teriyaki sauce, 1 cup of cooked whole wheat couscous, and ½ cup of green peas

Evening snack: ½ cup of pear slices tossed with ½ ounce of blue cheese or Brie

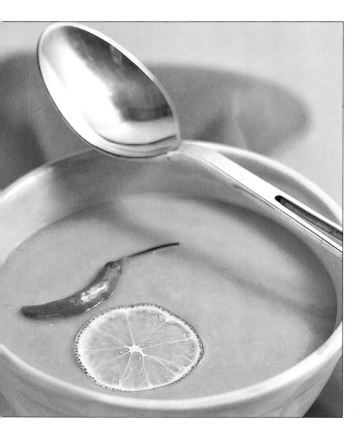

Day's total: 1,586 calories, 46 grams of fat, 15 grams of saturated fat, 28 grams of fiber, and 1,803 milligrams of sodium

Positively Delicious

The following sampling of recipes for the Positive-Eating Plan will help you develop a sense of a healthy new eating approach that stars vegetables, fruits, whole grains, and legumes. These foods supply ample doses of vitamins, minerals, and fiber, all of which are known to promote good health. Plus, they are naturally low in calories and fat, which will help you lose weight without even trying.

Carrot Soup with Lime and Chiles

Hands-on time: 10 minutes
Total time: 35 minutes

1 tablespoon olive or canola oil

1 large onion, finely chopped

2 large cloves garlic, chopped, or 1 tablespoon prepared chopped garlic

½ pound peeled, ready-to-eat baby carrots

½ cup uncooked instant brown rice

2 cans (14½ ounces each) fat-free, reduced-sodium chicken broth

1 cup water

½ teaspoon salt

2 tablespoons chopped green chiles + additional for garnish (optional)

Juice of 1 lime (about 2 tablespoons)

¼ cup plain yogurt (optional)

Chopped fresh cilantro (optional)

Chapter 5

Dine Out without Filling Out

Think of restaurant menus as made-to-order rather than off-the-rack.

Our fast-paced lifestyles have fueled a demand for both comfort and convenience, and eating out delivers both. If you're like the average woman, you eat out about four times a week, mostly lunch. The problem is, dining out can also mean filling out.

Researchers at the University of Memphis found that women who ate out at least six times a week consumed 288 more calories and 19 more grams of fat a day than those who ate out five times a week or less. That easily translates to 25 extra pounds a year! It's scary, but hardly surprising.

When we step into a restaurant, we enter the Fat Zone, a seductive netherworld of jalapeño poppers; baby back ribs; and creamy, cheesy, oily sauces. To make things worse, restaurant portion sizes are mammoth, an obvious fact to those of us who routinely undo the top button of our jeans once we climb back into our cars.

But take heart. When it comes to dining out, there are plenty of ways to keep fun on the menu without padding your waistline.

Your Eating-Out Action Plan

If you put certain skills and strategies into action, it's possible to eat healthfully and enjoyably in 99 percent of restaurants, says Hope Warshaw, R.D., a nutrition consultant in Washington, D.C., and author of *The Restaurant Companion: A Healthier Guide to Eating Out*.

These skills share one common theme: Master the menu. The strategies below can help you make healthier choices in any eatery.

Skill #1: Practice portion control. We're suckers for all-you-can-eat buffets, 50-item salad bars, and entrées preceded by words like jumbo, grande, supreme, king-size, and feast. To control portion sizes from the get-go, you need only three magic words: "Wrap it up."

"Even the finest restaurants are happy to wrap leftovers," says Penny Pollack, dining editor of *Chicago Magazine*. "There's nothing low-class or embarrassing about it. And if you know you can eat the rest of the meal tomorrow, you'll be more likely to stop eating when you're full tonight."

Try these portion-control tactics as well.

• Ask if you can order half-, lunch-, or appetizer-size portions.

• Make a meal of appetizers or side dishes. Mix and match dinner salads, broth-based soups

1-MINUTE FAT BURNER

Blot the fat. You can take off about 1 teaspoon of oil—or 40 calories and 4.5 grams of fat—from two slices of pizza.

(like vegetable, beef vegetable, or chicken noodle), or appetizer portions of pasta, for instance.

• If you're a regular at several different restaurants, scrutinize the menus at each and choose three nutritious, low-fat, low-calorie dishes. Then when you visit these restaurants again, order these healthy choices automatically, without even opening the menu. When you get bored, select another few healthy items and rotate among your favorites.

Skill #2: Speak up—nicely. "Making special requests is essential to getting foods as you want them," says Warshaw. And chefs are usually glad to oblige. A survey by the National Restaurant Association found that more than 9 out of 10 restaurants would, upon request, serve sauce or salad dressing on the side, prepare foods with vegetable oil instead of butter, and broil or bake an entrée rather than fry it.

Generally, customers make these basic types of requests: asking the chef to omit high-fat, high-calorie ingredients such as cheese, bacon, and sour cream; requesting the substitution of one side dish for another (like steamed veggies or a salad instead of french fries); and asking that a dish be prepared with less fat (cut back on the butter or oil; hold the mayo or cheese).

Skill #3: Learn to say "fat" in five languages. We all know that french fries, Buffalo wings, and bacon cheeseburgers are fat bombs. But the word "fat" comes in many guises: "chimichanga" at Mexican restaurants, "carbonara" at Italian eateries, "crispy" at Chinese places, and "biryani" at Indian restaurants. Wherever you dine, items that you order baked, broiled, grilled, poached, roasted, or steamed are typically lower in fat and calories.

Chinese Food

Whether you order from the take-out joint down the street or dine at a cozy little place with cloth napkins, Chinese food can be either a healthy eater's nightmare or a dream come true, says Warshaw. It depends on what you order and how much you eat.

The trick is to eat like a woman from the Chinese countryside: lots of steamed rice and steamed fresh vegetables and small amounts of meat, poultry, or seafood.

Perhaps your biggest challenge, though, is to minimize the tremendous amount of fat used in Americanized Chinese cuisine. It's best to avoid deep-fried items, says Warshaw.

If you watch your salt intake, leave the soy sauce on the table. Even the low-sodium kind packs 600 milligrams per tablespoon.

Top picks: Wonton or hot-and-sour soup; steamed dumplings; steamed or stir-fried veggies, seafood, or chicken; and dishes prepared with a light wine or lobster sauce.

Oil slicks: The deep-fried, crispy noodles served as an appetizer; egg rolls; fried dumplings; spare ribs; Peking duck; dishes prepared with cashews or peanuts; and entrées described as "crispy" or "sweet and sour."

American Food

There's nothing wrong with eating at diners or steakhouses; many of us love the convenience and casual atmosphere. Of course, there's a reason that diners are affectionately called greasy spoons, but if you order carefully and make special requests, healthy choices are plentiful, says Warshaw. Just be sure to steer clear of most "diet plates," she cautions. "They became popular in the 1950s, when protein was in and carbohydrates were out. They're usually a hamburger or

---

Who's Doing the Cooking These Days?

In 1970, we spent 26 percent of our food dollars on dining out. By 1996, the number climbed to 39 percent.

- On an average day in 1998, 21 percent of U.S. households used some form of takeout or delivery.
- Almost 50 billion meals are eaten in restaurants and school and work cafeterias each year.
- The average annual household expenditure for food away from home in 1997 was $1,921, or $768 per person.

When You Can't Resist, Have Some Fun

Does eating healthy mean you should never order dessert? Or french fries? Or spare ribs? Not at all. Sometimes, you just have to have your favorites without feeling like a nutritional criminal. Here are a few tips on how to indulge wisely.

Go big on the grease. If you really want something fried, choose large-size items—a breast of chicken instead of five or six chicken fingers, or seven or eight steak fries instead of 20 or more thin french fries. The smaller items have more total surface area, so they absorb more oil, making them higher in fat and calories, says Gayle Reichler, R.D., a registered dietitian and consultant in New York City and author of *Active Wellness: Feel Good for Life*.

Learn to share. Order one serving of a favorite high-fat food, such as french fries or spare ribs, and share it with everyone at the table, says Julie Waltz Kembel, a behavioral therapist specializing in weight loss in Tucson and author of *Winning at the Weight and Wellness Game*.

Have a doughnut. Despite their fat-filled image, you can get fewer calories and less fat if you order a glazed yeast doughnut (170 calories, 9 grams of fat) with your coffee instead of almost any kind of muffin, including banana nut (360 calories, 15 grams of fat), chocolate chip (400 calories, 17 grams of fat) and bran (390 calories, 12 grams of fat).

Think small and satisfying for dessert. It may be easier than you think to skip the gooey treats—and about 80 percent of us do when we eat out. But if you really can't resist ending on a sweet note, Kembel suggests ordering two or three chocolate mints with your coffee or tea.

Declare a holiday twice a month. Letting yourself enjoy an occasional free meal is as much a part of slimming down as that high-fiber cereal stocked in your pantry. "Anticipating something special is the spice of life for all of us," notes Kembel. And there has to be a place for the occasional extravagance in your thinner lifestyle.

Rather than depriving yourself of birthday cake or a romantic dinner on your anniversary, plan to indulge. Eat whatever you want in whatever quantity you want, but limit it to twice a month, says Kembel.

Think of this little piece of contrarian advice as a way to strike a balance between your desire to eat a healthy, low-fat diet and your need to have a little fun.

cottage cheese, with maybe some canned fruit or crackers."

The whole idea behind steakhouses, however, is to serve "mammoth" portions of meat. Some serve 24- and even 96-ounce steaks (that's 6 pounds!), slabs large enough to choke Fred Flintstone. Make sure you stick to one serving of meat, which is about 3 ounces, and ask to have the extra fat trimmed away before cooking. Few steakhouses offer a cut of meat that weighs less than 8 ounces, so be prepared to split it or ask that half be wrapped before it even hits the table, says Audry Triplett, head chef at Gibsons, a popular steakhouse in Chicago.

Enjoy your 3-ounce portion of beef with a cup of broth-based soup or a salad, a side dish of steamed vegetables, and a plain baked potato. By the way, do ask if a small potato is available. Many restaurants present you with a spud that's the size of a Nerf football. If they can't fulfill your request for a smaller potato, you can share with a friend or wrap part of it to go, says Triplett.

Top picks: Peel-and-eat shrimp; shrimp cocktail; fresh fruit cup (in juice, not syrup); dinner salads with low-fat dressing on the side. Fresh veggies from the all-you-can-eat salad bar. Broth-based soups; a small hamburger; a bacon, lettuce, and tomato sandwich (mayonnaise on the side); a large Greek or spinach salad (dressing on the side); or a turkey, chicken, roast beef, or ham sandwich on whole grain bread with let-

---

1-MINUTE FAT BURNER

Order fish. Varieties rich in omega-3 fatty acids, such as tuna, mackerel, cod, and salmon, may help you drop pounds by improving fat metabolism. Overweight people who ate a reduced-calorie diet that included fish every day lost about 20 percent more weight than those on a fish-free diet.

---

tuce, tomato, and mustard, barbecue sauce, or low-fat dressing. In 3-ounce portions, lean cuts of beef such as top sirloin (229 calories, 14.2 grams of fat) or tenderloin (258 calories, 18.6 grams of fat); a well-trimmed lamb chop (172 calories, 8.31 grams of fat); or a pork loin chop (178 calories, 8.2 grams of fat).

Oil slicks: Deep-fried appetizers; creamy soups such as New England clam chowder; melts; club sandwiches; Reuben sandwiches; jumbo burgers; baby back ribs; macaroni and potato salads; and most platters, which are typically served with french fries and creamy coleslaw.

Italian Food

Whether you dine at a candles-in-the-Chianti-bottle trattoria or a four-star hideaway, the rule is this: Follow the path of least mozzarella. While most Italian food is heavily Americanized, there are usually several healthy choices, says Maria Giordano Lupo, chef at Va Tutto restaurant in New York City. Here's what to look for.

Top picks: Grilled meat, poultry, or fish; pasta with red or white clam sauce; pasta pomodoro (sautéed fresh tomatoes, basil, garlic, and a small amount of olive oil); and pasta primavera without cream sauce. Risotto and polenta are also good picks, as long as they're made with spices and vegetables rather than butter and cheese. Risotto is made with rice, and polenta is a dish made with cooked cornmeal.

If you're ordering pizza, ask for extra marinara sauce and half the cheese. Add some toppings and you'll barely notice the difference. Request a thin-crust pie rather than Sicilian or deep-dish. And obviously, order your pie piled high with veggies rather than sausage or pepperoni.

Oil slicks: Antipastos with cheeses, olives, and salami; anything carbonara (cream, eggs, cheese, and bacon); and anything parmigiana (breaded, fried, and smothered in mozzarella). And watch out for the garlic knots; they're dripping in oil or melted butter. Leave them in the basket or send them away with the waiter.

Indian Food

If you like your food spicy, chances are, you enjoy Indian cuisine. If you're watching your weight, there's even more to love, like the fact that Indian food is based on healthy complex carbohydrates, particularly legumes like chickpeas and lentils, and veggies such as spinach, eggplant, potatoes, and peas.

The downside is the fat used to prepare many of these dishes. Many appetizers are deep-fried, and vegetables and meats are typically fried or sautéed in the Indian butter called *ghee*.

Still, "most Indian restaurants provide plenty of choices for the low-fat diner," says Priya Kulkarni, an Indian cooking instructor and coauthor of *Secrets of Fat-Free Indian Cooking*. "As a general rule, avoid dishes that have the words

'butter' or 'coconut' in their menu descriptions. And stay away from those that are cooked in a creamy sauce and those that contain large amounts of nuts." Here are her thumbs-up and thumbs-down selections.

Top picks: Mulligatawny soup; naan, roti, and chapati breads, which are baked rather than fried; dals (legume dishes; choose those without cream); chana (chickpea curry); kachumbars (vegetable salads); raitas (salads with a tart yogurt dressing); and dishes described on the menu as masala (a combination of spices with sautéed tomatoes and onions) or tandoori (seasoned meat, poultry, or fish roasted in a clay oven).

Oil slicks: Samosas (deep-fried pastry filled with vegetables or meat); puri (a puffy, deep-fried bread); and entrées described as biryani, malai, or korma, which are heavy on the oil or cream.

Mexican Food

We love Mexican food. Unfortunately, we love it prepared American-style, which means knee-deep in fat, especially at chain restaurants and Mexican fast-food places.

In those establishments, the perfectly healthy staples of Mexican cuisine—corn, beans, and tomatoes—are smothered with cheese and sour cream or heaped into deep-fried shells. "You won't find a salad served in a deep-fried tortilla shell in Mexico," notes Warshaw. And we won't even mention the basket of deep-fried tortilla chips the waitress sets on the table as soon as you take your seat—and keeps refilling.

Yet it is possible to go Mexican and eat healthfully. The goal is to bring this fare back to its healthier, more nutritious roots, says Felipe Gaytan, executive chef at Via Reál, a Mexican restaurant in Irving, Texas.

Top picks: Grilled chicken or fish; items wrapped in a soft flour tortilla, such as fajitas and burritos; and *pescado Veracruzana* (fish in Veracruz sauce). The Veracruz sauce contains olive oil, grilled onions, green olives, and capers, which give it a tangy flavor. Other options: *mole pollo* (boned chicken breast served in a hot and spicy sauce) and *camarones de hacha* (shrimp

Eat Soup—And Drop up to 10 Pounds in a Year

By this time next year, you could be wearing your "skinny" slacks, just by starting one meal a day with a broth-based soup. Why? A new study suggests that soup can help you eat 100 fewer calories a day, which means you could drop 10 pounds this year even if all the other factors in your diet stay constant.

Respected diet expert Barbara Rolls, Ph.D., professor at the Pennsylvania State University in University Park and coauthor of *Volumetrics: Feel Full on Fewer Calories*, recently tested 24 college women at the university. Shortly before lunch, on 3 different days, the women were asked to eat either a small portion of chicken rice casserole, the same-size portion of casserole plus a 10-ounce glass of water, or a large bowl of chicken rice soup that consisted of the casserole ingredients mixed with 10 ounces of water. The calories in all three appetizers were the same—270.

Seventeen minutes later, the women were presented with a buffet lunch of sliced ham and cheese, kaiser rolls, romaine lettuce, tomato and cucumber slices, chips and pretzels, strawberry yogurt, cookies, and chocolate bars—and told to eat as much as they wanted.

Dr. Rolls found that after the women ate the chicken rice casserole—either alone or with a glass of water—they went on to choose lunches that averaged nearly 400 calories. But after they ate the chicken rice soup, they chose lunches that averaged only about 300 calories.

The women who ate the chicken rice soup didn't make up the extra calories later in the day, either. At a buffet dinner, they chose food averaging about the same calories as the casserole groups. Breakfasts were about the same size, too. So for the entire day, the soup group ate 100 fewer total calories.

Breakfast: A Reason to Stay Home

Eat breakfast out, and you can easily blow a day's worth of fat, not to mention 1,000 calories, by 10:00 A.M. Sure, you know that eggs are high in cholesterol and bacon isn't diet food. But who would have guessed that pancakes with butter or margarine and sausage have as much artery-clogging power as a fast-food burger and french fries?

When researchers at the University of Memphis compared the nutrient quality of meals at home with meals at restaurants, breakfast came up the big loser. People who ate breakfast out consumed more fat, more calories, and half the fat-fighting fiber that people who ate breakfast at home did.

The bottom line: If you're trying to start your day on the right foot, nutritionally speaking, don't go out for breakfast, says Linda Eck Clemens, R.D., Ed.D., a professor of clinical nutrition at the University of Memphis and a registered dietitian.

Of course, it is possible to get a healthy breakfast when you eat out. Go for hot or cold cereal, fruit, juice, plain toast or English muffins, a small bagel, or some fat-free yogurt. Many restaurants also offer egg substitutes. Combine them with hash browns and plain toast, and you have a pretty decent breakfast.

sautéed in a red and green tomato sauce). Enjoy them with a side of rice and pinto, kidney, or black beans with no added fat.

Or increase your options by ordering à la carte. For example, make a meal of a bowl of black bean soup, a dinner salad dressed with salsa or low-fat dressing on the side, and one bean, seafood, chicken, or beef burrito or fajita.

Oil slicks: Deep-fried tortilla chips; anything topped with cheese, sour cream, or guacamole; refried beans (commonly fried in lard); chimichangas (deep-fried flour tortillas filled with meat and cheese); the Mexican sausage called chorizo; and deep-fried taco-shell bowls.

Chapter 6

Do All Those Wacky Diets Really Work?

Surprise! You'll find a grain of truth in most of them.

Got a health problem? Check the Internet or watch the next talk show, and you'll find a wacky diet to cure it. "Just stop eating the wrong stuff and start my diet," their creators assert, "and you'll lose your allergies! Overcome fatigue! Live longer! Shed pounds effortlessly!"

The theories behind some of these diets are so intriguing (for example, can your blood type really dictate what you should eat?) that it's natural to wonder: Could they work? You might be especially curious if you've known someone who's tried one of these diets and is convinced that it helped.

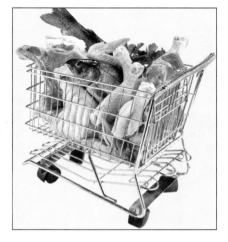

"Unless you're a scientist with courses in biology and physiology, it's hard to sort fact from fiction," says Judith Stern, Sc.D., professor of nutrition and medicine at the University of California, Davis, and vice president of the American Obesity Association.

So we asked the experts. Surprisingly, they gave us reasons why each of the following diets has both hype *and* hope.

Food-Combining Diet

Two books currently on the market that espouse versions of the old diet idea of combining foods are *Suzanne Somers' Eat Great, Lose Weight* and Harvey and Marilyn Diamond's *Fit for Life*.

The claim behind it: This type of diet is based on the belief that many health problems occur because we eat foods in the wrong combinations. If you eat the wrong foods together at the same meal, you confuse your body into producing the wrong digestive enzymes. That leaves undigested food to rot and turn into poisons in your intestines.

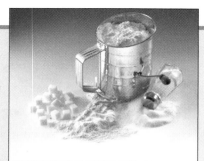

Should You Beware "The Five White Dangers"?

According to the Hallelujah Diet found on the Internet, "The Five White Dangers" are salt, sugar, white flour, dairy foods, and meat (it contains white fat). Eliminate these, the Hallelujah Diet claims, and you'll lose weight and fight off a slew of chronic diseases.

There's a grain of truth hidden in this drastic claim. When it comes to salt, sugar, white flour, and meat (but not dairy foods), there's reason to believe that cutting down may in fact improve your health—though for reasons other than those described in the Hallelujah Diet.

To cut down on salt, sugar, and white flour, you'll need to cut down on processed foods, which are a source of too many empty calories in most diets. As for meat, people who eat less of it do lower their risk of chronic disease, says registered dietitian Cyndi Thomson, R.D., Ph.D., a research instructor at the University of Arizona College of Public Health in Tucson, whose specialty is cancer prevention. In place of processed foods and meat, you'll be eating more vegetables, fruit, and whole grains, which is right in line with *Prevention*'s diet recommendations.

But we don't recommend eating less dairy. Dairy foods are most people's major source of calcium. If you do cut down, eat high-calcium foods such as tofu set with calcium, calcium-fortified citrus juice, and calcium-fortified soy milk.

The promise: If you stop combining the wrong foods, you'll start digesting your meals fully. The result? You'll lose weight, increase energy, and even reverse food allergies.

What you eat: Eat fruit only by itself, and only in the morning. Eat protein and fat with vegetables, but not with carbohydrates. Eat carbohydrates with vegetables only, never with fat or protein.

The experts' view: In fact, few foods occur as pure protein, carbohydrate, or fat, as this diet implies. Most foods are a mix, making it virtually impossible to keep components separate. Whole wheat bread, for example, isn't pure carbohydrate, it's also 15 percent protein and 14 percent fat.

What's more, it's impossible to confuse your digestive enzymes. Each has just one job to do. In a lock-and-key fashion, each enzyme pairs with the correct substance and severs its chemical bond. "Fortunately, your digestive system is quite capable of making multiple enzymes in just the right mix for what you're eating at the time," says registered dietitian Cyndi Thomson, R.D., Ph.D., a research instructor at the University of Arizona College of Public Health in Tucson.

The grain of truth: Strict rules about what-goes-with-what almost automatically limit the size of your meals. This diet emphasizes low-calorie fruits and vegetables (no soft drinks or cupcakes on the "yes" list). Eating smaller meals and lots of produce are both good ways to lose weight. "That's why you may lose weight practicing food combining," says Dr. Thomson.

What to watch out for: Short term, you'll do okay on this diet. But the structure limits your intake of calcium-rich dairy foods

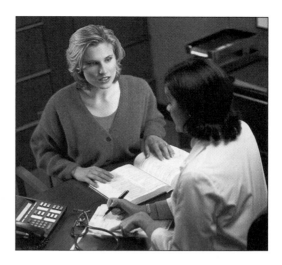

Unless you're a scientist with courses in biology and physiology, **it's hard to sort fact from fiction**.

while opening the door to foods high in saturated fat. That's bad for your bones, blood pressure, and heart. And if you have a life-threatening food allergy, beware: The only way to control it is to avoid the offending food.

‖ Blood-Type Diet

This diet originated with the book *Eat Right for Your Type* by Peter D'Adamo, N.D. Another version is *The Answer Is in Your Bloodtype* by Steven Weissburg, M.D.

The claim behind it: Our different blood types—O, A, B, and AB—evolved in response to the varying environments and diets faced by prehistoric man. Knowing your blood type can tell you what's the best diet (and exercise) for your digestive tract and immune system.

The promise: If you follow the right diet and exercise for your blood type, you can stay healthy, live longer, and achieve your ideal weight.

What you eat: If your blood type is O, your Stone Age hunter ancestry means that you need lots of meat and intense exercise, but few grains and little dairy.

Blood type A indicates that you are descended from prehistoric farmers and require a vegetarian diet because you don't produce enough hydrochloric acid to digest meat. Gentle forms of exercise, such as yoga or meditation, are best for you.

Blood type B points to your nomadic ancestry and suggests that you need mostly dairy and a little meat, but no chicken and few grains. You need moderate exercise.

If you have blood type AB, you represent a merging of types A and B and need a varied diet that emphasizes seafood, dairy, wheat-free grains, and soy foods. Yoga and mild aerobics are the best types of exercise for you.

The experts' view: "This is pure pseudoscience," says Dr. Stern. "The blood-type theory has never been tested clinically with results published in peer-reviewed journals." One clue that something's amiss: The idea that some people need less exercise than others based on blood type flies in the face of everything we know.

Another red flag is the suggestion that people with type-A blood don't have enough hydrochloric acid. It's true that some people's stomachs produce less hydrochloric acid, but that comes with age, not blood type. And the problem with too little hydrochloric acid is that you can't absorb enough vitamin B_{12}, not that you can't digest protein.

The Best and Worst High-Protein Diets

Prevention says that the healthiest weight-loss diet is one that's based on plant foods—about 15 percent protein, 25 percent fat, and 60 percent mostly unprocessed carbohydrates (vegetables, fruits, and whole grains).

To be sure, all the high-protein diets are based on bogus science—the erroneous idea that carbohydrates make you fat. You think you're losing weight because you're following a "scientific" plan that focuses on "protein blocks" or "reward meals." But you're really losing weight because you're eating fewer calories, not because you're eating fewer carbohydrates. It's as simple as that.

To follow the moderate high-protien diets, however, you cut back on starchy carbohydrates and sweets, substituting meat and tons of vegetables in their place. For most people, that means trading in nutrient-empty white flour and sugar for nutrient-laden protein and produce—a huge step in the right direction. And if it helps you achieve a healthy weight, fantastic!

We surveyed an array of popular high-protein diets to zero in on what we think is the best—and the worst. We've also included a fix to make the best even better.

BEST:
SUGAR BUSTERS!

Food focus: Lean protein; legumes; low-fat dairy foods; high-fiber fruits, vegetables, whole grain breads and cereals

Calorie control: Small portions, no seconds

Considered the enemy: All sugars, sweets, corn, carrots, beets, white potatoes, rice, bread

Sample Menu

- Breakfast: Orange juice, wheat bran cereal, fresh strawberries, fat-free milk
- Lunch: Lean roast beef on whole wheat bread with lettuce and tomato
- Snack: Kiwifruit, 6 walnut halves
- Dinner: Turkey breast, baked sweet potato, steamed green beans
- Dessert: 2 thin slices of cheese

Risks: You get unnecessarily obsessed with every grain of sugar. A few healthy foods, such as carrots, are demonized. This diet is a little low in calcium, folate, and iron.

Benefits: Provides a great array of healthy choices, including whole grains. Rich in fiber, vitamins A and C, the B vitamins, and zinc.

The fix: Choose calcium-fortified orange juice and take a daily multivitamin/mineral supplement.

WORST:
DR. ATKINS'S NEW DIET REVOLUTION

Food focus: Bacon, fried eggs, fried pork rinds, high-fat cheese, butter, cream

Calorie control: Limits carbohydrates to 20 grams (the amount in one hot dog bun) to provoke ketosis, which inhibits hunger

Considered the enemy: Most breads and cereals, fruit, and starchy vegetables are severely limited. Milk and sugars are forbidden.

Sample Menu

- Breakfast: Fried eggs with sugar-free sausage
- Lunch: Bacon cheeseburger (no bun), small tossed salad
- Dinner: Shrimp cocktail with mustard and mayo, clear consomme, steak, tossed salad with dressing, diet Jell-O with artificially sweetened heavy cream

Risks: Bad breath, constipation, and elevated cholesterol. Oozes saturated fat and limits many foods known to protect your health.

Benefit: Rapid weight loss.

The fix: Honor your body enough to choose a different diet.

The Healthy Way to Go High-Protein

If you decide to follow a high-protein diet, here are rules to help you use—but not abuse—the staying power of protein.

- Have your doctor test your kidney function before you start a high-protein diet to make sure that your kidneys are healthy.
- Choose a diet that maximizes your intake of high-fiber, brightly colored veggies—and be sure to eat all of the veggies that are allowed.
- Select a diet that emphasizes meats and poultry that are low in saturated fats. Trim the fat, and don't char your meats.
- Pick a diet that includes at least 50 grams of carbohydrates daily to prevent ketosis (a potentially dangerous, abnormal metabolism state).
- Drink 8 cups of fluid daily to help your kidneys.
- Select whole grain breads and cereals when possible.
- Opt often for soy-based foods, legumes, and fish for your protein choices.
- Choose low-fat dairy foods and calcium supplements to reach 1,500 to 2,000 milligrams of calcium daily.
- Take a standard (not high-potency) multivitamin/mineral supplement daily.

And just as a practical matter: How would you feed a family of four with different blood types?

The grain of truth: Limited food choices automatically cut calories, so you may lose weight as long as you can stick with the limited food choices.

What to watch out for: No matter what your blood type, this diet sets you up to exclude too many foods. You lose fiber and vitamin E by excluding grains; fall short of carotenoids and phytochemicals when skipping vegetables; and miss out on calcium when you don't do dairy.

The "Mayo Clinic" Diet

Before you start this diet, be aware that it neither originated at the Mayo Clinic nor is it approved by the famed medical center. But does it work?

The claim behind it: If you eat only certain combinations of foods, you'll burn more fat. Adding some grapefruit burns fat even faster.

The promise: On this diet, you can eat as much as you want and still lose weight permanently.

What you eat: At every meal, eat half a

Weight Loss
HELP OR HYPE?

Do Weight-Loss Supplements Ever Work?

Should you try to speed up weight loss with a natural supplement that promises to control your appetite, make you burn more calories (without exercise), and prevent extra calories from being converted to body fat?

Those are the powerful promises being made for two supplements: pyruvate, which is a natural by-product of energy production in the body, and garcinia (*Garcinia cambogia*), a tropical fruit that is rich in the compound hydroxycitric acid.

The Evidence

Much of the research testing pyruvate's ability to aid weight loss comes from Ronald Stanko, M.D., associate professor of surgery at the University of Pittsburgh Medical Center. Dr. Stanko holds the patent for the use of pyruvate in weight loss. He has published two human studies showing that supplementing ultra-low-calorie diets (500 to 1,000 calories a day) with more than 20 grams of pyruvate a day (an extremely high dose, about 10 times the recommended amount) resulted in very small increases in weight loss—an average of 2 to 3 pounds over 3 weeks—compared to those who got placebos. According to Dr. Stanko, such small differences can make a big difference over time, especially for weight gain caused by middle-age spread. He currently recommends 3 to 5 grams of pyruvate a day for gradual weight loss.

The evidence for garcinia, however, is less impressive. One well-controlled study done by Steven Heymsfield, M.D., of St. Luke's–Roosevelt Obesity Research Center in New York City, found that 1.5 grams of hydroxycitric acid from garcinia given for 12 weeks to overweight men and women had no effect on weight or fat loss. So far, only studies in rats have suggested that garcinia may reduce appetite.

The Bottom Line

When put in perspective, both pyruvate and garcinia lose their quick-fix appeal. More well-controlled studies need to be done before the weight-loss promises of garcinia can be taken seriously.

Pyruvate may provide an extra nudge to weight-loss attempts when it's combined with exercise and a reduced-calorie diet, but it won't effortlessly melt away the extra pounds.

Caution: If you have an ulcer, you should avoid taking pyruvate on an empty stomach.

grapefruit. The rest of your menu is as follows: breakfast is two eggs and two slices of bacon; lunch is a salad with dressing and meat; and dinner is a salad with dressing, meat, and a nonstarchy vegetable cooked in butter. Drink eight glasses of water and one glass of fat-free milk or tomato juice a day. Avoid most dairy, starchy fruits and vegetables, and grains. Do this for 12 days, then take 2 days off and eat anything you want. Repeat as needed.

The experts' view: "Clearly, there is no science to support this," says Tammy Baker, R.D., a Phoenix-based spokesperson for the American Dietetic Association. "And grapefruit is not magic." Alas.

The grain of truth: Why do some people lose weight on this diet? That's easy. A low-calorie menu plan puts your appetite on autopilot for a while, and restricting food choices (did you notice that there are no desserts?) limits your calories. Men especially seem to find the high-protein diets such as this one filling and satisfying. "But people eventually get bored," says Baker. "And pretty soon, you're staring wistfully at your spouse's baked potato."

What to watch out for: If you don't choose lean meats, eating all those foods high in saturated fat can raise your risk of heart disease. Plus, calcium is low to absent, notes Baker. Any high-protein diet is hard on the kidneys and should definitely be avoided if you are at risk of kidney disease (if you have diabetes, for example).

1-MINUTE FAT BURNER

Trigger your body's own "appetite shut-off switch." Eat 2 to 3 ounces of protein at lunch (a small chicken breast), and you're likely to eat 31 percent fewer calories at dinner.

The Bottom Line

Compelling passion is the hallmark of most "miracle diet" creators, and often their enthusiasm is impressive, if not their science. Luckily, following these plans for a short time won't be fatal, and some people say that they do feel better. What's interesting is that each diet has lessons that can make anyone healthier, from cutting down on sweets to eating more low-calorie vegetables to making meals smaller if you need to lose weight.

Since these diets so often result in weight loss, it would be fair to ask this question: What's the harm as long as I can drop a few pounds? "Overweight people think diets such as these can't hurt," says Dr. Stern. "But they can, because they prevent you from seeking a reasonable approach to weight management that you can sustain."

Another critical drawback: If you do manage to stick with one of these diets for the long term, you'll be setting yourself up for nutrient deficiencies. Many women already face a calcium crisis, getting only half of what they need, and all of these fad diets would make that worse.

Here's our advice: For a nutrient-packed eating plan designed to maximize good health and control your weight, follow the plan explained.

Chapter 7

Now You're Cooking!

Delicious, healthy recipes make it easy to eat right for life.

A s the saying goes, you are what you eat. And the dishes you prepare at home can give you a big boost—by revving up your energy, giving you the glow of good health, preventing disease, and helping you lose weight.

You know that you'll look and feel great if you eat right, but you may still feel skeptical about making healthy eating a regular part of your life. That may be because you've bought into these myths about healthy eating.

Myth #1: Healthy eating means that I can't eat red meat ever again. Never say never. The keys are moderation and choosing wisely. Certain cuts of pork and beef have nutritional profiles comparable to that of a skinless chicken breast.

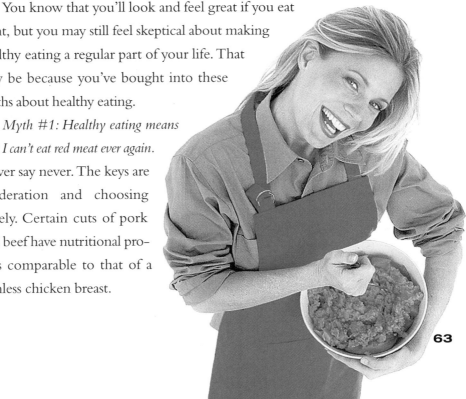

Myth #2: Healthy eating means that I'll have to give up my favorite foods. The recipes in this chapter should help dispel this myth. They show how to cook delicious dishes for breakfast, lunch, and dinner that are low in fat and high in the nutrients that help prevent disease.

Myth #3: Healthy foods take longer to cook. Nobody has hours to spend in the kitchen. The recipes in this chapter are as quick to prepare as many of the old standbys you've been making for years. Healthy cooking can be quick and easy.

Myth #4: I can never eat dessert again. If you've tried to deny yourself this universal pleasure, you know how hard it is. And you don't have to! The keys here, too, are moderation and choosing wisely. This chapter provides recipes for scrumptious desserts that can fit into healthy meals.

Why Cook This Way?

Healthy cooking pays off in many ways. Here are some big ones.

You can eat more. When you cut back on fat, you can eat a greater amount of food. That's because fatty foods are a denser source of calories than healthier, carbohydrate-rich and protein-rich foods.

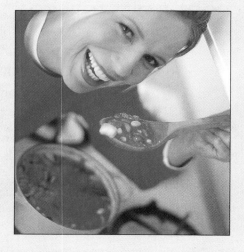

You'll lose weight. One of the best ways to lose a few pounds is with a healthier diet. Not only will you look and feel better, but losing weight also cuts your risk for many illnesses, including heart disease, high blood pressure, diabetes, stroke, and certain cancers.

You'll love the taste. If you eat right, you may find yourself loving food more than ever. "We've found that food with less fat allows people to more fully enjoy the experience of eating," says John La Puma, M.D., director of the CHEF (Cooking Healthy Eating Fitness) pilot study at Alexian Brothers Medical Center in Elk Grove, Illinois. After 10 weeks of eating lower-fat food, subjects in this study reported an increase in their range of flavor appreciation. "There is a shift from appreciating mainly the full, rich, heavy, round flavors in fat to appreciating the bright, clean, citrusy, fresh flavors of foods with less fat. Eating less fat may actually broaden your palate and your enjoyment of food," says Dr. La Puma.

Apple Skillet Cake

Hands-on time: 15 minutes
Total time: 1 hour and 15 minutes

1 tablespoon butter or margarine
3 apples, peeled and sliced
2 tablespoons packed light brown sugar
½ teaspoon ground cinnamon
½ cup raisins
¾ cup unbleached or all-purpose flour
⅓ cup sugar
⅛ teaspoon salt
1½ cups 1% milk
2 eggs
1 egg white
2 teaspoons vanilla extract

Preheat the oven to 375°F.

Melt the butter or margarine in a 10" oven-proof skillet over medium-high heat. Add the apples. Cook for 2 minutes, or until slightly softened. Add the brown sugar, cinnamon, and raisins. Cook for 5 minutes, turning occasionally, or until the apples are tender when pierced with a knife.

Meanwhile, in a large bowl, combine the flour, sugar, and salt.

In a medium bowl, whisk together the milk, eggs, egg white, and vanilla extract. Add to the flour mixture. Whisk just until smooth. Pour into the skillet with the apple mixture.

Bake for 40 to 45 minutes, or until golden brown and puffed. Remove to a rack to cool for 5 minutes.

To serve, cut into wedges. With a pancake turner, lift each wedge and turn, apple side up, onto a plate.

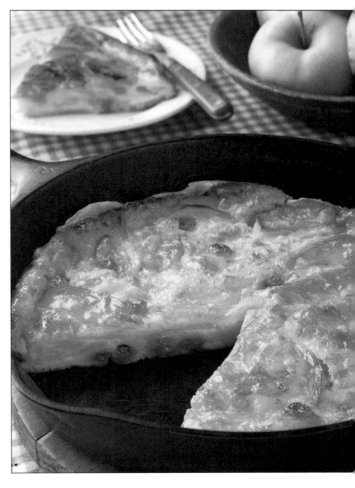

Makes 6 servings
Per serving: 270 calories, 7 g protein, 51 g carbohydrates, 5 g total fat, 2 g saturated fat, 78 mg cholesterol, 2 g dietary fiber, 114 mg sodium

South-of-the-Border Frittata

Hands-on time: 5 minutes
Total time: 20 minutes

1 egg
5 egg whites

1 can (15 ounces) black beans, rinsed and drained

1 cup corn kernels

⅔ cup (2½ ounces) shredded low-fat Monterey Jack cheese

¾ teaspoon chile powder

1 bunch scallions, sliced

¼ cup (2 ounces) fat-free sour cream

¼ cup salsa

In a medium bowl, whisk together the egg, egg whites, beans, corn, Monterey Jack, and chile powder. Set aside.

Coat a large nonstick skillet with nonstick spray. Add the scallions. Coat lightly with nonstick spray. Cook, stirring, over medium heat for 1 to 2 minutes, or until wilted.

Add the reserved egg mixture to the skillet. Cook, stirring occasionally, for 7 to 8 minutes, or until the eggs are set on the bottom. Reduce the heat to low. Cover and cook for 4 to 5 minutes, or until the eggs are set on the top.

To serve, cut into wedges and top with the sour cream and salsa.

Makes 4 servings

Per serving: 229 calories, 20 g protein, 27 g carbohydrates, 6 g total fat, 3 g saturated fat, 67 mg cholesterol, 7 g dietary fiber, 751 mg sodium

Cornmeal Flapjacks

Hands-on time: 25 minutes

Total time: 25 minutes

1 cup cornmeal

¾ cup unbleached or all-purpose flour

1 teaspoon baking soda

½ teaspoon salt

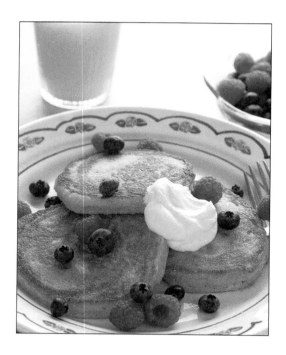

1¼ cups buttermilk

1 egg

2 tablespoons maple syrup

1 tablespoon vegetable oil

Preheat the oven to 200°F. Coat a baking sheet with nonstick spray.

In a large bowl, combine the cornmeal, flour, baking soda, and salt.

In a medium bowl, combine the buttermilk, egg, maple syrup, and oil. Beat with a fork or whisk until blended. Add to the flour mixture. Stir until a smooth batter forms.

Coat a large nonstick skillet with nonstick spray. Warm over medium heat. Pour the batter by ¼ cupfuls into the skillet. Cook for 2 minutes, or until tiny bubbles appear on the surface and the edges begin to look dry. Flip the pancakes. Cook for 1 to 2 minutes, or until golden on the bottom. Transfer the pancakes to the prepared baking sheet. Place in the oven to keep warm.

Coat the skillet with nonstick spray. Repeat with the remaining batter to make a total of 15 pancakes.

Makes 5 servings

Per serving: 248 calories, 8 g protein, 45 g carbohydrates, 4 g total fat, 1 g saturated fat, 44 mg cholesterol, 3 g dietary fiber, 557 mg sodium

Club Sandwiches

Hands-on time: 15 minutes
Total time: 15 minutes

Lemon-Caper Mayonnaise

½ cup low-fat mayonnaise

1 teaspoon lemon juice

2 teaspoons drained capers, coarsely chopped

Sandwiches

12 thin slices multigrain bread, toasted

½ pound cooked skinless chicken breast, sliced

2 ounces alfalfa sprouts

⅓ English cucumber, thinly sliced

1 large tomato, cut into 8 slices

8 slices turkey bacon, cooked

4 leaves lettuce

To make the lemon-caper mayonnaise: In a small bowl, combine the mayonnaise, lemon juice, and capers.

To make the sandwiches: Place 4 of the bread slices on a work surface. Spread 2 teaspoons of the lemon-caper mayonnaise on

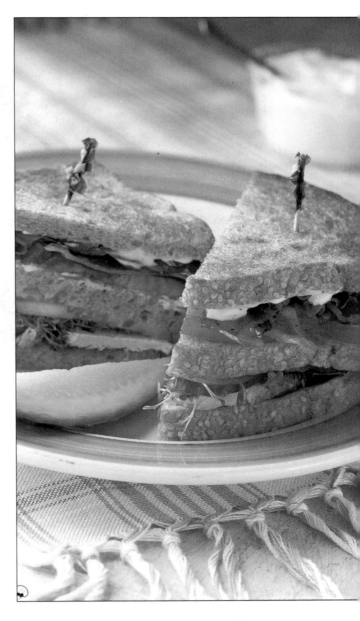

each slice. Top with layers of chicken, alfalfa sprouts, and cucumber.

Spread 4 of the remaining bread slices each with 2 teaspoons of lemon-caper mayonnaise.

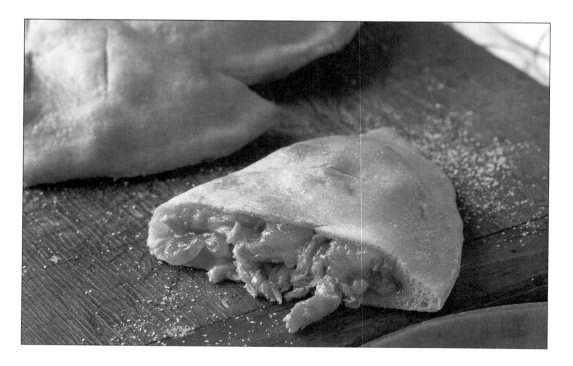

Place, mayonnaise side up, on the 4 sandwiches. Top with layers of tomato, bacon, and lettuce.

Spread the remaining 4 bread slices with the remaining lemon-caper mayonnaise. Place, mayonnaise side down, on top of the sandwiches. Cut in half diagonally. Secure with toothpicks.

Makes 4 servings

Per serving: 349 calories, 29 g protein, 41 g carbohydrates, 9 g total fat, 2 g saturated fat, 79 mg cholesterol, 10 g dietary fiber, 1,060 mg sodium

Note: Although this sandwich is relatively high in sodium, traditional club sandwiches can contain up to three times as much sodium in a serving. If sodium is a concern for you, omit the bacon and use only 2 slices of bread per sandwich. For further fat reduction, replace the turkey bacon with Canadian bacon or a soy-based imitation bacon.

Barbecue Chicken and Cheddar Calzones

Hands-on time: 25 minutes
Total time: 50 minutes

1　tablespoon cornmeal

1　large onion, halved and thinly sliced

¾　pound boneless, skinless chicken breast, cooked and shredded (see note)

1　cup barbecue sauce

2　tubes (10 ounces each) refrigerated pizza dough

1　cup (4 ounces) shredded low-fat Cheddar cheese

1　egg white, lightly beaten with 1 teaspoon water

Preheat the oven to 375°F. Coat a baking sheet with nonstick spray. Sprinkle with the cornmeal.

Coat a medium nonstick skillet with nonstick spray. Set over medium heat. Add the onion. Cook, stirring occasionally, for 5 to 7 minutes, or until soft. Add the chicken and barbecue sauce. Stir to mix.

Turn the dough out onto a lightly floured work surface. Divide into 4 equal pieces. Roll 1 piece of dough into a 7" circle. Place ½ cup of the chicken mixture on 1 side of the circle, spreading to within 1" of the edge. Sprinkle with ¼ cup of the Cheddar. Brush the edges of the crust with some of the egg-white mixture. Fold the circle in half. Pinch the edges to seal. Repeat with the remaining dough and filling to make a total of 4 calzones.

Transfer to the prepared baking sheet. Brush the calzones with the remaining egg-white mixture. With a sharp knife, make 3 small slashes in the top of each calzone.

Bake for 20 to 25 minutes, or until the crusts are golden brown. To serve, cut each calzone in half.

Makes 8 servings

Per serving: 357 calories, 24 g protein, 51 g carbohydrates, 5 g total fat, 2 g saturated fat, 39 mg cholesterol, 3 g dietary fiber, 673 mg sodium

Note: Cook the chicken on a broiler or in a large nonstick skillet coated with nonstick spray. Broil or cook over medium-high heat for 5 to 7 minutes per side, or until a thermometer inserted in the thickest portion registers 160°F and the juices run clear. Remove the chicken to a plate. Set aside for 5 minutes. Pull into shreds with a fork.

Chicken Fajitas

Hands-on time: 15 minutes
Total time: 30 minutes

2   tablespoons lime juice

2   tablespoons fat-free reduced-sodium chicken broth

2   cloves garlic, minced

½   teaspoon dried oregano

⅛   teaspoon salt

1   pound boneless, skinless chicken breast, cut into thin strips

8   flour tortillas (6" diameter)

1   medium red onion, sliced into thin wedges

2   green and/or yellow bell peppers, cut into ½"-wide strips

2   cups finely shredded green leaf lettuce

½   cup (2 ounces) shredded low-fat Cheddar or Monterey Jack cheese

½   cup salsa

½   cup (4 ounces) fat-free sour cream

In a medium bowl, combine the lime juice, broth, garlic, oregano, and salt. Add the chicken. Toss to coat evenly. Place in the refrigerator to marinate for 20 minutes.

Preheat the oven to 350°F. Wrap the tortillas in foil. Bake for 10 minutes, or until warmed through. Turn the oven off, but do not remove the tortillas.

Meanwhile, coat a large nonstick skillet with nonstick spray. Add the onion and bell peppers. Coat with nonstick spray. Cook, stirring occasionally, over medium-high heat for 6 to 8 minutes, or until crisp-tender. Remove to a bowl. Cover loosely with foil.

vith nonstick spray. Remove
ᴇ marinade. Place in the
ᴍarinade. Cook, stirring, for
ᴇ juices run clear. Return
...ᴏ ᴏnion and bell peppers to the pan. Toss for
1 minute to heat through.

Arrange the tortillas on 4 plates. Spoon the
chicken mixture over the tortillas. Top with lettuce, cheese, salsa, and sour cream.

Makes 4 servings

Per serving: 420 calories, 46 g protein, 40 g
carbohydrates, 7 g total fat, 3 g saturated fat, 106
mg cholesterol, 14 g dietary fiber, 741 mg sodium

Baked Potato Skins

Hands-on time: 5 minutes
Total time: 1 hour and 20 minutes

1 large russet potato

2 large sweet potatoes

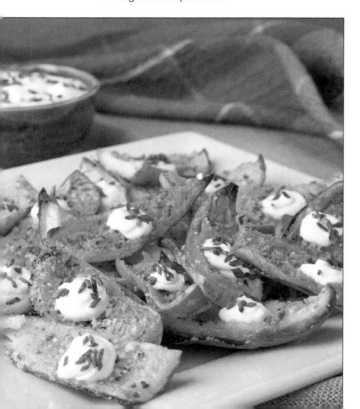

½ cup (2 ounces) grated Parmesan cheese

1 tablespoon chopped fresh parsley

1 teaspoon dried basil leaves

½ teaspoon garlic powder

½ teaspoon salt

½ cup (4 ounces) fat-free sour cream

2 tablespoons chopped fresh chives or scal-
lion greens

Preheat the oven to 425°F. Line a baking
sheet with foil. Pierce each potatoe a few times
with a fork. Place on the prepared baking sheet.
Bake for 50 to 60 minutes, or until easily pierced
with a fork. Remove and allow to cool slightly.

Meanwhile, in a small bowl, combine the
Parmesan, parsley, basil, garlic powder, and
salt.

When the potatoes are cool enough to
handle, quarter them lengthwise. Scoop out the
flesh, leaving a ¼"-thick shell. Reserve the flesh
for another use. Cut the strips in half crosswise.
You should have 24 wedges. Place on the foil-
lined baking sheet. Coat both sides with nonstick spray. Sprinkle with the Parmesan mixture.

Bake for 10 to 12 minutes, or until golden
brown. To serve, top with dollops of sour
cream. Sprinkle with the chives or scallions.

Makes 8 servings

Per serving: 114 calories, 5 g protein, 19 g
carbohydrates, 2 g total fat, 1 g saturated fat, 5
mg cholesterol, 3 g dietary fiber, 280 mg sodium

Nachos

Hands-on time: 10 minutes
Total time: 20 minutes

1 small onion, chopped

3 cloves garlic, chopped

1 can (19 ounces) cannellini beans, rinsed and drained

1 teaspoon ground cumin

¼ teaspoon salt

2 roasted red peppers, chopped

4 plum tomatoes, chopped

½ cup frozen corn kernels, thawed

2 scallions, sliced

2 tablespoons chopped fresh cilantro or parsley

1 tablespoon lime juice

6 ounces small baked tortilla chips

1½ cups (6 ounces) shredded low-fat Monterey Jack cheese

Preheat the oven to 350. Coat a 13" × 9" baking dish with nonstick spray.

Coat a medium nonstick skillet with nonstick spray. Set over medium heat. Add the onion and garlic. Cook, stirring often, for 5 minutes, or until soft. Add the beans, cumin, and salt. With the back of a spoon, coarsely mash the beans. Remove from the heat.

Meanwhile, in a medium bowl, combine the peppers, tomatoes, corn, scallions, cilantro or parsley, and lime juice.

Spread the chips in the prepared baking dish. Dot with dollops of the bean mixture and the pepper mixture. Sprinkle with the Monterey Jack.

Bake for 5 to 7 minutes, or until the cheese has melted.

Makes 8 servings

Per serving: 227 calories, 13 g protein, 34 g carbohydrates, 5 g total fat, 3 g saturated fat, 15 mg cholesterol, 5 g dietary fiber, 604 mg sodium

Thai Shrimp Bisque

Hands-on time: 15 minutes
Total Time: 40 minutes

2 teaspoons butter or margarine

1 small onion, finely chopped

1 carrot, finely chopped

1 rib celery, finely chopped

1 clove garlic, minced

¾ pound large shrimp, peeled, deveined, and cut into thirds

2 cans (14½ ounces each) fat-free reduced-sodium chicken broth

2 cups water

1 can (15 ounces) diced tomatoes, drained

⅓ cup long-grain white rice

1½ teaspoons paprika

¼ teaspoon salt

1 cup reduced-fat coconut milk

2 teaspoons grated fresh ginger

1–2 tablespoons lime juice

Melt the butter or margarine in a Dutch oven over medium heat. Add the onion, carrot, celery, and garlic. Cook, stirring often, over medium heat for 5 minutes. Add the shrimp. Cook, stirring, for 2 to 3 minutes, or until the shrimp are opaque. Remove the shrimp and set aside.

Add the broth, water, tomatoes, rice, paprika, and salt. Bring to a boil. Reduce the heat to medium-low. Partially cover and cook for 20 minutes, or until the rice is tender. Return half of the shrimp to the pot.

Transfer the soup to a food processor or blender, working in batches if necessary. Process until pureed. Set a fine strainer over the pot. Pass the soup through the strainer, pressing with the back of a spoon. Discard the pulp. Add the reserved shrimp, coconut milk, and ginger. Cook over low heat for 4 to 5 minutes, or until heated though. Season with the lime juice to taste.

Makes 6 servings

Per serving: 194 calories, 15 g protein, 18 g carbohydrates, 4 g total fat, 2 g saturated fat, 84 mg cholesterol, 2 g dietary fiber, 443 mg sodium

Minestrone

Hands-on time: 15 minutes
Total time: 45 minutes

1 tablespoon olive oil

1 onion, chopped

2 large cloves garlic, chopped

2 carrots, chopped

2 ribs celery, chopped

2 teaspoons Italian seasoning

1 can (48 ounces) fat-free reduced-sodium chicken broth or vegetable broth

1 can (15 ounces) diced tomatoes

¾ pound green beans, cut into 1" lengths

1 large zucchini, cut into ¼" cubes

¼ Savoy or green cabbage, thinly sliced

½ cup ditalini or other small pasta

¼ teaspoon salt

1 can (19 ounces) cannellini or red kidney beans, rinsed and drained

Warm the oil in a Dutch oven set over medium heat. Add the onion and garlic. Cook, stirring often, for 3 minutes, or until the onion starts to soften. Add the carrots, celery, and Italian seasoning. Cook for 3 minutes, or until the carrots are crisp-tender. Add the broth. Increase the heat to high and bring to a boil. Reduce the heat to medium-low. Cook for 10 minutes, or until the carrots are almost tender. Add the tomatoes (with juice), green beans, zucchini, cabbage, pasta, salt, and beans. Simmer for 10 to 12 minutes, or until the pasta is cooked and all the vegetables are soft.

Makes 8 servings

Per serving: 202 calories, 15 g protein, 27 g carbohydrates, 4 g total fat, 2 g saturated fat, 5 mg cholesterol, 9 g dietary fiber, 372 mg sodium

Stir-Fried Beef and Broccoli

Hands-on time: 30 minutes
Total time: 35 minutes

¼ cup fat-free reduced-sodium chicken broth

3 tablespoons dry sherry or fat-free reduced-sodium chicken broth

½ cup orange juice

1 teaspoon grated orange peel (optional)

2 tablespoons soy sauce

1 tablespoon grated fresh ginger

1 tablespoon sugar

2 teaspoons cornstarch

1 teaspoon toasted sesame oil

½ teaspoon crushed red-pepper flakes

1 pound beef sirloin, trimmed of all visible fat and cut into ¼"-thick strips

⅔ cup white rice

2 teaspoons vegetable oil

1½ pounds broccoli florettes

1 bunch scallions, cut in ¼" diagonal slices

3 cloves garlic, chopped

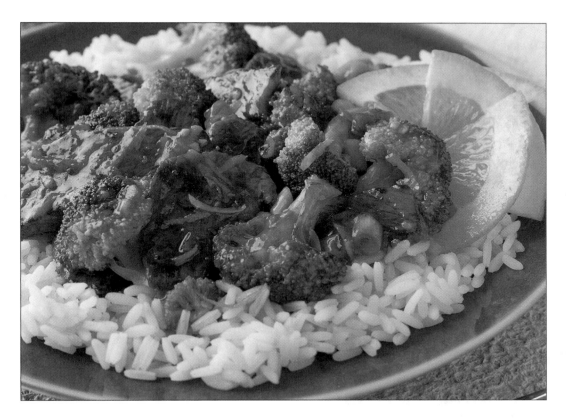

In a medium bowl, combine the broth, sherry or broth, orange juice, orange peel (if desired), soy sauce, ginger, sugar, cornstarch, sesame oil, and red-pepper flakes. Stir to mix. Add the beef, tossing to coat evenly. Allow to marinate for 20 minutes.

Meanwhile, prepare the rice according to package directions.

Heat a large skillet over medium-high heat. Coat with 1 teaspoon of the vegetable oil. Lift the beef from the marinade into the skillet. Reserve the marinade. Cook the beef, stirring constantly, for 2 to 3 minutes, or until browned. Remove to a plate.

Add the remaining 1 teaspoon vegetable oil to the skillet. Add the broccoli, scallions, and garlic. Cook, stirring occasionally, for 2 minutes. Add 2 tablespoons water. Cover the pan and cook for 1 to 2 minutes, or until the broccoli is crisp-tender. Add the reserved marinade. Cook, stirring constantly, for 3 minutes, or until the mixture boils and thickens slightly.

Reduce the heat to medium-low. Return the beef to the pan. Cook, stirring, for 2 minutes, or until the beef is heated through. Serve over the rice.

Makes 4 servings

Per serving: 412 calories, 32 g protein, 47 g carbohydrates, 10 g total fat, 3 g saturated fat, 71 mg cholesterol, 4 g dietary fiber, 363 mg sodium

Orange Roughy Veracruz

Hands-on time: 15 minutes
Total time: 35 minutes

4   orange roughy or red snapper fillets
    (4 ounces each)

1   tablespoon lime juice

1   teaspoon dried oregano

2   teaspoons olive oil

1   onion, chopped

1   clove garlic, minced

1   can (15 ounces) Mexican-style diced
    tomatoes

12 pimiento-stuffed olives, coarsely chopped

2   tablespoons chopped parsley

Preheat the oven to 350°F. Coat an 8" x 8" baking dish with nonstick spray. Place the fillets in the baking dish. Sprinkle with the lime juice and oregano. Set aside.

Warm the oil in a medium skillet set over medium heat. Add the onion and garlic. Cook, stirring occasionally, for 5 to 6 minutes, or until soft. Add the tomatoes, olives, and parsley. Cook, stirring occasionally, for 5 minutes, or until thickened. Spoon over the fillets. Cover tightly with foil.

Bake for 18 to 20 minutes, or until the fish flakes easily.

Makes 4 servings

Per serving: 163 calories, 18 g protein, 12 g carbohydrates, 4 g total fat, 1 g saturated fat, 23 mg cholesterol, 2 g dietary fiber, 503 mg sodium

Chocolate Chippers

Hands-on time: 20 minutes
Total time: 55 minutes

2¼ cups unbleached or all-purpose flour

¼   cup cornstarch

1   teaspoon baking soda

½   teaspoon salt

¼   cup butter or margarine, softened

2   ounces reduced-fat cream cheese, softened

¾   cup granulated sugar

¾   cup packed light brown sugar

1   egg

1   egg white

1   teaspoon vanilla extract

¾   cup chocolate chips

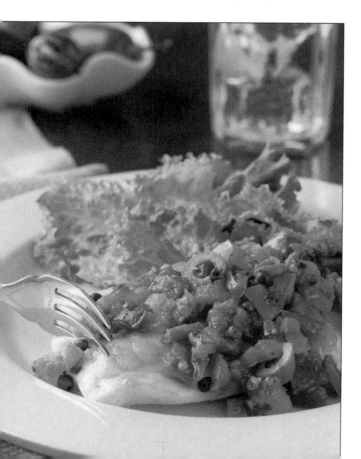

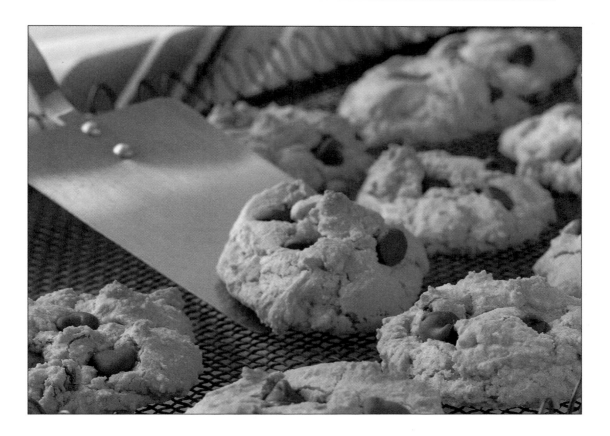

Preheat the oven to 375°F. Lightly coat a baking sheet with nonstick spray.

In a medium bowl, combine the flour, cornstarch, baking soda, and salt.

In a large bowl, combine the butter or margarine and cream cheese. With an electric mixer on medium speed, beat for 1 minute, or until smooth. Add the granulated sugar and brown sugar. Beat until light and creamy. Add the egg, egg white, and vanilla extract. Beat until smooth. Reduce the mixer speed to low. Add the flour mixture in 2 additions, beating just until combined. With a spoon, stir in the chocolate chips. Drop the dough by rounded teaspoonfuls onto the prepared baking sheet.

Bake for 9 to 12 minutes, or until golden. Remove the cookies to a rack to cool. Repeat until all the cookies are baked.

Makes 40

Per cookie: 90 calories, 1 g protein, 16 g carbohydrates, 3 g total fat, 1 g saturated fat, 6 mg cholesterol, 0 g dietary fiber, 72 mg sodium

Plum-Blueberry Cobbler

Hands-on time 20 minutes
Total time: 1 hour

8 plums, quartered

1 pint fresh or frozen blueberries

½ cup + 4 teaspoons sugar

 2 tablespoons + 1 cup unbleached or all-
   purpose flour

 ¾ teaspoon baking powder

 ⅛ teaspoon salt

 ½ cup buttermilk

 1 egg white, lightly beaten

1½ tablespoons vegetable oil

Preheat the oven to 375°F. Coat an 8" × 8" baking dish with nonstick spray.

In a large bowl, combine the plums, blueberries, ½ cup of the sugar, and 2 tablespoons of the flour. Pour into the prepared baking dish.

In a medium bowl, combine 3 teaspoons of the remaining sugar, the baking powder, salt, and the remaining 1 cup flour.

In a small bowl, combine the buttermilk, egg white, and oil. Pour into the medium bowl with the flour mixture. Stir until a thick batter forms. Drop the batter in tablespoonfuls on top of the fruit. Sprinkle with the remaining 1 teaspoon sugar.

Bake for 35 to 40 minutes, or until golden and bubbly. Remove to a rack to cool. Serve warm or at room temperature.

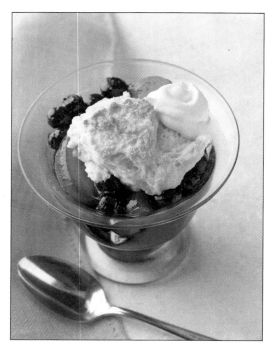

Makes 8 servings

Per serving: 238 calories, 4 g protein, 50 g carbohydrates, 4 g total fat, 0 g saturated fat, 1 mg cholesterol, 3 g dietary fiber, 107 mg sodium

LIFESTYLE RESTYLE

She Slimmed Down with Weekend Splurges

During the week, Helene Gullaksen is spartan about her food choices. But when the weekend arrives, she lets loose. "I eat whatever I please," says the 35-year-old resident of Stockholm, Sweden. "I shop for special treats, I go out for dinner with my husband, and sometimes I pig out on pizza."

Relaxing her strict dietary rules on weekends keeps Gullaksen from feeling deprived. It also helped her lose 50 pounds.

Like many women, Gullaksen didn't have a weight problem until after her two pregnancies. "With my first baby, I went from 132 pounds to 180 pounds," she recalls. "I managed to lose about 38 pounds before I got pregnant again." After giving birth to her second child, she kept right on gaining, eventually reaching 190 pounds.

As much as Gullaksen wanted to unload the extra pounds, she recoiled at the thought of dieting. "I enjoy eating, and I didn't want to feel deprived," she explains. So she made a deal with herself: If she ate healthfully during the week, she'd allow herself to splurge on weekends.

Gullaksen follows a weekday diet that is quite austere, limiting the number of calories that she consumes. Her breakfast typically consists of a whole grain roll with olives and sun-dried tomatoes. For lunch, she chooses between a low-calorie frozen entrée and a selection of buffet items from a restaurant near her workplace. "I don't even look at the 'bad' foods," she says. "I just fill my plate with beans, fresh vegetables, and fresh fruits." At dinnertime, she prepares a healthy meal for her family, then serves herself half-portions of whatever they're having.

Though Gullaksen still faces temptations during the week, knowing that she can splurge on weekends gives her incentive to stay true to her weekday diet. "When I get a craving during the week, I tell myself, 'It's not the last time that I'll have an opportunity to eat this food,'" she says.

Gullaksen's weekdays-on, weekends-off eating plan—and walking whenever she gets a chance—helped her go from 190 pounds to 135 pounds in just 9 months. She has maintained her weight since 1997.

Her weekend splurges are more low-key than they used to be. In fact, she no longer experiences cravings for candy or ice cream, two of her former favorite foods. "I try to listen to my body and give it what it asks for, no more and no less," she says.

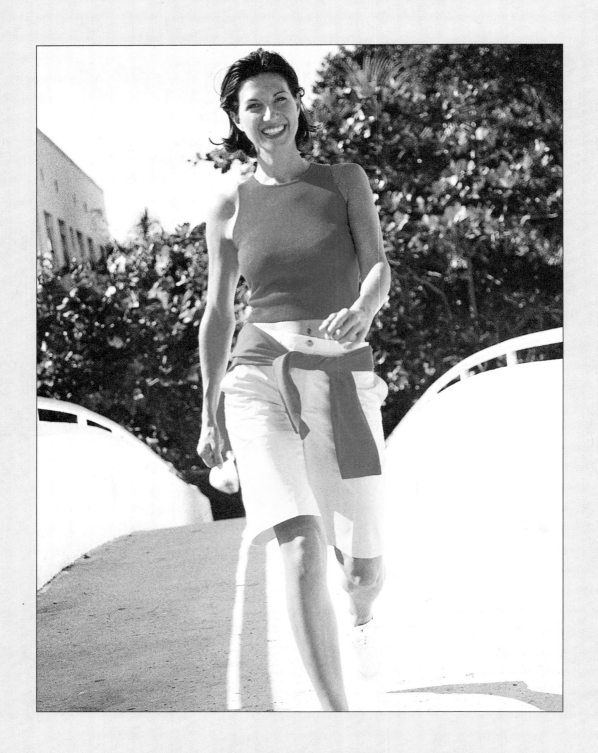

Part Three

Fitting In
Fitness

Chapter 8

How Fit Are You?

Tailor your fitness program based on these simple tests.

Being in shape means being able to enjoy daily life to the fullest. It means bounding up stairs, hustling down the block, and hoisting groceries without feeling tired or weak. What's the best way to get back in youthful shape? Exercise, of course. But it's a whole lot easier to reach your fitness goals if you know where to begin.

That's where fitness testing comes in. By checking a few important aspects of fitness such as balance, stamina, strength, and flexibility, you can find out where you've maintained your fitness over the years, and where you haven't. That way you can tailor a fitness program to your unique exercise needs and start stepping confidently toward a fitter, stronger you.

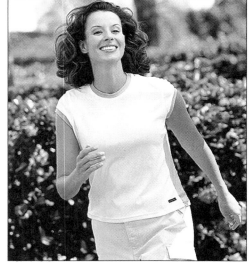

Try This at Home

Intimidated by the thought of taking a fitness test? Don't be. Unlike the ones you took in your high school gym class, no one is watching or judging you. And the truth is, you're probably in better shape than you think.

"People often assume that because they're heavier than the models they see in magazines, they must be in terrible shape, but that's not usually true," says Joyce A. Hanna, associate director of the health improvement program at Stanford University. "Usually, folks find that they're a little weak in a couple of areas, but pretty well-off in others. It's very empowering to know where you rank against the norm, and that with just a little effort, you can really improve."

With that in mind, try the following fitness tests and see where you rank. Some of these tests are a little tough; some are just fun. Then try the suggestions for improvement, and come back again in a few months and take the tests again.

We'll bet that you not only score higher the second time around but you'll also start enjoying life a little more, as everyday tasks get easier to do and you find yourself with energy to burn.

Good luck!

Can You Take a Bow?

Few of us think of flexibility when we think of fitness. But we should, says Michelle L. Edwards, a health educator at the Cooper Institute for Aerobics Research in Dallas and a certified personal trainer.

"Tight, inflexible muscles make daily living harder," Edwards says. "We stop being able to tie our shoes without sitting down. We're more likely to pull muscles and get injured. Flexible muscles just make you feel better."

The toe-touch test. Stand with your feet shoulder-width apart. Keeping your legs straight (but not locking your knees), bend over from the waist and reach toward the floor. Note how close your fingertips get to the ground.

How Did You Do?

If You Reached	Your Score Is
The floor, palms down	Excellent
Your toes	Good
Your ankles	Fair
Above your ankles	Too tight

Bend better. It takes only about 10 minutes a day to improve flexibility and make those muscles long and limber. Try the stretch routine "Limber Up!" on page 112, and you'll be touching those toes in no time.

Are You Strong to the Core?

Strong trunk or "core" muscles, such as your abdominals, make everyday tasks from vacuuming the floor to working long hours at a desk job easier to do because they can support your body better, says Edwards. "Strong abdominal muscles are also important for helping prevent back pain," she says. Here's how to test yours.

The situp test. Lie on your back with your knees bent and your feet flat on the floor. Place your fingers behind your head. Have a friend hold down your feet, or secure them under a piece of furniture. Set a timer or have your friend time you for 1 minute.

Do as many full situps as you can. For a situp to count, you have to bring your elbows up to touch your knees, and lower yourself back down so that your shoulders touch the floor.

Keep your arms loose. Do not pull on the back of your head or neck. To avoid straining your head and neck muscles, you might try crossing your arms lightly across your chest, placing the tips of your fingers at the side of your head, or holding your arms straight out. Your head should stay straight in line with your back throughout the exercise.

How Did You Do?

If You Did This Many Situps		Your Score Is
age 20–29	44–50	Excellent
	38–43	Good
	32–37	Fair
	24–31	Poor
age 30–39	35–41	Excellent
	29–34	Good
	25–28	Fair
	20–24	Poor
age 40–49	29–37	Excellent
	24–28	Good
	20–23	Fair
	14–19	Poor
age 50–59	24–29	Excellent
	20–23	Good
	14–19	Fair
	10–13	Poor
age 60+	17–27	Excellent
	11–16	Good
	6–10	Fair
	3–5	Poor

Build a stronger core. The recipe for building a strong core starts with strong abdominal muscles. You can improve yours quickly and easily by doing exercises such as abdominal crunches. As a bonus, your tummy will feel thinner, too!

Your Best Balancing Act

Our balance often gets shakier as we get older, mostly because we stop using it, says John Yetter, M.D., medical director at SSM Rehab Sports Medicine in St. Louis. "All the running and jumping we do as kids requires a lot of balance. Staying active as adults can help us keep it. And that means less falls as we get older."

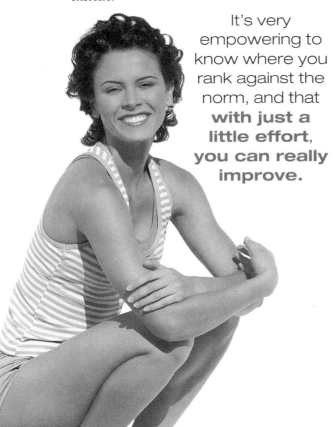

It's very empowering to know where you rank against the norm, and that **with just a little effort**, you can really improve.

The single leg stand. Stand on your strongest leg (usually the same side as your dominant hand).

Raise the opposite leg so that your knee is out in front of you, while keeping the knee of the supporting leg slightly bent. You can flex the raised knee about 30 degrees, if that's more comfortable.

Keep your arms down by your sides and see how long you can balance.

How Did You Do?

If You Balanced	Your Score Is
More than 30 seconds	Excellent
21–30 seconds	Good
11–20 seconds	Fair
10 or fewer	Poor

Be better balanced. Strong muscles build better balance, says Edwards. "Basic weight training to strengthen your legs, back, and torso can sharpen your balance and improve your strength dramatically." Try the 10 simple exercises in "The Fat-Fighting Workout" on page 115.

Your Upper-Body Oomph

"Americans are getting very, very weak in their upper bodies," says Hanna. Good upper-body strength makes all the fun stuff in life, such as gardening and home projects, a whole lot easier, she says. "And it's particularly important for women to help prevent osteoporosis." Here's a quick way to check yours.

The pushup test. Get in a pushup position with your legs bent so that you're

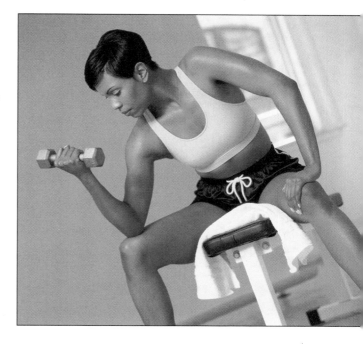

Upper body strength is particularly important for women to help **prevent osteoporosis**.

supporting your weight with your hands and your knees. Your body should form a straight line from your head to your knees. This is a modified pushup position for women, since they are built with less upper-body mass than men.

Set a timer for 1 minute, or have someone time you. Keeping your back straight, lower your chest to about 3 inches (the size of a fist) off the floor. Push back up. That's one pushup. Do as many as you can in 1 minute. You can rest between reps if you need to, but only in the "up" position, not on the floor.

How Did You Do?

If You Did This Many Pushups		Your Score Is
age 20–29	36–44	Excellent
	30–35	Good
	23–29	Fair
	17–22	Poor
age 30–39	31–38	Excellent
	24–30	Good
	19–23	Fair
	11–18	Poor
age 40–49	24–32	Excellent
	18–23	Good
	13–17	Fair
	6–12	Poor
age 50–59	21–30	Excellent
	17–20	Good
	12–16	Fair
	6–11	Poor
age 60+	15–19	Excellent
	12–14	Good
	5–11	Fair
	2–4	Poor

Build a better upper body. Pushups are one of the best exercises for building upper-body strength, says exercise physiologist and certified personal trainer Ann Marie Miller, fitness director of New York Sports Clubs in Manhattan. Try doing two sets of 8 to 12 repetitions twice a week.

‖ How's That Tiger in Your Tank?

With all of the elevators and escalators in office buildings and shopping malls, it's easy to lose those little bursts of power for bounding up stairs or striding up steep hills. But good anaerobic fitness (the kind of fitness you use for short bursts of speed and power) means you can sprint for a bus and run up a flight of stairs without heaving for breath and feeling ready to drop.

"When you improve in this category, you really start feeling younger. You have a spring in your step again," says Dr. Yetter.

The stair-climb test. Walk up 30 to 40 steps without stopping. (If you aren't near a long flight of stairs, you can walk up and run down a small flight of fewer steps several times.) You can hold the handrail if you need to.

Wait 60 seconds, then take your pulse for 10 seconds, and multiply it by six. (It's easiest to take your pulse by lightly placing two fingers on the side of your neck.)

How Did You Do?

If Your Pulse Was	Your Score Is
Less than 90	Excellent
90–100	Good
101–120	Fair
Above 120	Poor

Power up. Building stronger legs will help put more stride in your step. The chair squat exercise found on page 118 is a great place to start.

‖ Can You Shop 'til You Drop?

The walking test is one of the best tests of your aerobic fitness for everyday life, says Carla Sottovia, a certified exercise physiologist at the Cooper Fitness Center in Dallas. "You have to be able to walk to enjoy things like shopping and sightseeing," she points out. Plus, improving your aerobic fitness lowers your risk of heart disease.

The 1-mile walk test. Map out a flat 1-mile course. A ¼-mile walking track is ideal.

Warm up by walking leisurely for 3 to 5 minutes, then stretch gently.

Note the time on your watch (or start a stopwatch), and begin walking as quickly as you can without running, at a pace you can sustain for the entire course.

Check the time when you finish, cool down, and stretch.

1-MINUTE FAT BURNER

Retire the remote. You could easily burn 200 extra calories a day if you stop using the TV/VCR remote, garage door opener, electric can opener, riding mower, and other labor-saving devices.

Do the walk of life. "Walking still rules for aerobic fitness," says Dr. Yetter. "It's fun, it's easy to do, and it's natural." For tips on making your walking work for you, check out the advice in Walk Off Weight Your Way on page 101.

How Did You Do?

If You Finished in This Number of Minutes		Your Score Is
age 40 and under	13:30 or less	Excellent
	13:31–16:00	Good
	16:01–18:30	Average
	18:31–20:00	Below Average
	20:01 or more	Low
age over 40	14:30 or less	Excellent
	14:31–17:00	Good
	17:01–19:30	Average
	19:31–22:00	Below Average
	22:01 or more	Low

Chapter 9

Get Started in Three Simple Steps

Put your mind, body, and spirit in motion today!

For most folks, the hardest part about starting a fitness program is simply getting started. That's because they go into it as though it were an arranged marriage. They dread the thought of dragging themselves through activities they don't really enjoy day in and day out for the rest of their lives.

The truth is, if you start out right, your exercise program can be a longtime love affair that keeps you glowing for years to come. But first, you need to forget just about everything you've ever learned about exercising.

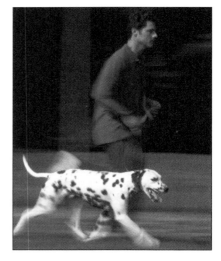

"In the past, we've made starting to exercise a daunting task," says Joyce A. Hanna, associate director of the health improvement program at Stanford University. "We made people get medical signatures, monitor their heart rates, take fitness tests, and so on. No wonder no one wanted to get started!"

You Can Start Today

Though some people should see their doctors before starting any kind of physical activity (see "Do You Need a Doc's Okay?"), for the most part, starting to exercise is no more difficult than putting down this book for 10 minutes and taking a quick walk around the block.

"Exercise doesn't have to be this big, long commitment that people think it is," says John Yetter, M.D., medical director at SSM Rehab Sports Medicine in St. Louis. "It should be about having some fun, like playing Frisbee with your kids or walking your dog through the park. We get to a point as adults where we get so tied up with the responsibilities of education, family, and career that we don't do these fun, active things anymore. Then we wake up one day and find that we can't button our pants, and we feel out

---

Do You Need a Doc's Okay?

Most healthy folks can roll right into a gentle fitness plan without checking with their doctors, says Joyce A. Hanna, associate director of the health improvement program at Stanford University. But if you've had health problems, you really should talk to your doctor before starting. You can use the following list as a guide, checking off the items that apply to you.

☐ You have a heart condition and have been advised to do only medically supervised physical activities.

☐ During or right after exercise, you frequently have pains or pressure in the left side of your chest or neck or in your left shoulder or arm.

☐ You have developed chest pain within the last month.

☐ You sometimes lose consciousness or fall over because you're dizzy.

☐ You feel unusually breathless after mild exertion.

☐ You're taking medication for blood pressure or a heart condition, or you have other physical problems, such as insulin-dependent diabetes.

☐ You have bone or joint problems that may get worse from physical activity.

☐ You are middle-age or older and have not been physically active before, and you're planning a relatively vigorous exercise program.

If you've checked one or more items, see your doctor before you start. If none of these apply to you, then you can get started.

of shape and old. It doesn't take more than 10 or 15 minutes—today—to break that cycle and start feeling younger and fitter again."

It's never too late to start. Even people in their nineties can get stronger, improve their moods, and reduce the risk for serious illnesses by putting more activity into their daily lives.

1. Jump-Start Your Mind

The biggest obstacle to a fit body is an unfit mindset. People often think that they're too busy or too out of shape to enjoy regular physical activity. So before working your body, you have to "train your brain," says certified international lifestyle fitness expert Lynne Brick, owner of Brick Bodies Health Clubs in Baltimore. "Once your thoughts start moving in a younger, more energetic direction, your body will quickly follow," she says.

Treat yourself like a friend. Your brain can be your best ally or your worst enemy when it comes to getting active, says Brick. "Make a decision to make it your friend," she says. "Whenever you start thinking, 'I'm old, I'm uncoordinated, I'm out of shape,' stop and ask yourself if you would tolerate a friend talking to you that way. Chances are that you wouldn't. Well, don't tolerate it from yourself either. Tell yourself, 'Okay,

I'm not where I want to be, but I have the ability to make myself better.' "

Don't make it a project. Once we become responsible adults, there's a tendency to become project-oriented: to make everything seem like a big deal, says Michael Gilewski, Ph.D., a clinical psychologist for postacute care services at Cedars-Sinai Medical Center in Los Angeles. "We make all these big decisions, like buying a car, switching jobs, or moving to a new home, that take detailed planning. Exercise isn't like that, yet many folks treat it the same way," he says. "Instead of making exercise yet another project, look at it as a break from your projects. Don't wait for the right time. You don't have to have all the right information or the right clothes. Just take a break right now and go do something."

Stop "working" out. Exercise will never be fun if you think of it as a dead-end job, says Laura Senft, a physical therapist at the Kessler Institute for Rehabilitation in West Orange, New Jersey. "Exercise shouldn't be work or drudgery. It should be fun and invigorating, more like play. So think of it as a play break for your mind, not a punishment session for your body."

Turn off the TV. The number one reason people give for not starting an exercise program is that they don't have the time. Don't believe it. "We all have the time; it all depends on how we use it," says Michael Bourque, certified personal trainer and personal training coordinator at the YMCA's Center for Health and Wellness in Oviedo, Florida.

"Sit down and figure out all that you do in a day," Bourque suggests. "That includes eating, sleeping, working, and miscellaneous activities.

Once your thoughts start moving in a younger, more energetic direction, **your body will quickly follow**.

Make Your Goals REAL

Setting goals is a great way to kick off a new fitness program. But many people choose goals that are fuzzy, such as, "I want to get in shape." This type of goal is tough to measure, so you'll never be sure if you're succeeding, says certified international lifestyle fitness expert Lynne Brick, owner of Brick Bodies Health Clubs in Baltimore.

When you're setting goals, she recommends using a mental checklist called REAL. This means making goals that are:

Realistic. If you're just getting started, don't expect to run 5 miles tomorrow. Instead, make it your goal to walk briskly for 20 minutes, 4 days a week, followed by longer sessions the following week.

Explicit. Be very specific about the goals you want to achieve. Tell yourself, for example, "I want to lower my body fat by 5 percent by the end of the year." This is much more explicit—and motivating—than just telling yourself, "I want to lose weight."

Action-oriented. Big goals are daunting. That's why it's often best to break down your "real" goal into smaller, "action-oriented" parts. For example, if your goal is to run a 5-K (about 3 miles), mentally break it down into ½- or ¼-mile increments. Achieving the parts makes it much easier to stay motivated for the whole.

Livable. Exercise is something you'll spend the rest of your life doing. So your goals should make you feel good, not miserable. Don't waste time forcing yourself to do things you don't enjoy. Find activities you truly like. That way, you'll always be motivated to keep doing them.

Inevitably, you'll find 2 to 3 hours that are unaccounted for. You can use that time to start an exercise program."

Promise yourself just 15 seconds. For some people, the idea of doing something physical for 45 minutes—or even 15 minutes—feels overwhelming. If that's the case, then promise yourself that you'll take just 15 seconds, says Al Secunda of Los Angeles, author of *Ultimate Tennis* and *The 15-Second Principle*. "You can do anything for 15 seconds. Promise yourself you'll do just 15 seconds' worth of abdominal crunches or squats," he says. "Some days, that may be all you do, and that's great. But most days, once you move for that 15 seconds, you'll find yourself revved up enough to do more."

2. Ready . . . Set . . . Go Slow!

One sure way to burn out on physical activity and end up feeling older rather than younger is to start out of the gate too quickly. It's important to ease into any activity. This allows your muscles to feel energized rather than wiped out and your mind to be invigorated rather than fatigued.

Rebuild your mind-body connection. Within your body, there are physical "memories" of running around, riding a bike, or playing hopscotch. But for most of us, these memories get buried beneath years of inactivity. "You can tap into them again by building up your activity level day by day," says Dr. Gilewski. "Today, go for a simple walk or ride around the neighborhood. It might feel a little awkward at first, but your body will start to remember what to do, and you'll be feeling great. Stop there, then go a little farther tomorrow. By the end of the month, you'll be back into the swing of things," he says. "In a few months, your body will think of exercise as a normal part of the day, and you'll start to crave it."

Warm up, cool down. Diving into any activity full blast puts undue strain on your muscles and tendons, and this almost guarantees that you'll stop your fitness program before it really gets going. Even if you're in the mood for a brisk jaunt around the park, start at a moderate pace for a few minutes, then pick up your speed, says Brick. Likewise, don't stop dead in your tracks when you're done. Slow to an easy walk and cool down before you stop.

Get comfortable. "You won't stay active very long if your feet hurt, you're overheated, or you're too cold," Dr. Gilewski says. "Try your new activity once or twice, then figure out what you need to be comfortable. If you're walking, for example, you should have comfortable walking shoes and clothes that keep you warm while letting your body breathe."

1-MINUTE FAT BURNER

Drop and do 10. Before you pry open that tub of ice cream, do 10 situps or pushups. Doing something physical can put you back in touch with your body—and your goals.

3. Boost Your Spirit

No matter how psyched up you feel about an exciting new physical activity, you are bound to hit some lulls soon after starting. It's just human nature, says Paul Konstanty, clinical supervisor and exercise therapist at the University of California OrthoMed Spine and Joint Conditioning Center in San Diego. You can avoid hitting a serious exercise slump by planning some rewards to acknowledge your efforts, boost your spirits, and keep your activity fresh.

Treat yourself. One of the best ways to stay motivated is to establish a reward system right off the bat, says Konstanty. "Promise yourself that if you are active so many days out of the upcoming month, you'll treat yourself to something nice. It could be a new pair of shoes or a night on the town," he says. "It'll give you something fun to look forward to, which is something we overlook all too often."

Plan some do-nothing days. Odd as it sounds, your fitness program will go longer and stronger if you occasionally blow it off and do nothing, says Dr. Gilewski. "Your muscles need days off now and then to recover," he explains. "Giving yourself permission to take a day to lounge around will make your fitness program seem less like a job, and this will leave you feeling even more energized to go back to it the next day."

Shoot for something. Kids play games and sports for a reason: They're not only fun but also rewarding and motivating. You can

Am I Too Sick to Exercise?

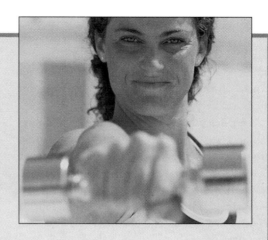

Fitness can be exactly what the doctor ordered," says Gloria Weinberg, M.D., chief of ambulatory medicine at Mount Sinai Medical Center in Miami Beach. "Or it can worsen the problem." What's best for your body? Check the chart below for some common ailments.

Ailment	Diagnosis	Rx	Warning
Common cold	Sniffly nose? Sore throat? Head cold? If you don't have a fever and your symptoms are at neck level or above, you can exercise.	Start working out at roughly 60 percent of your usual intensity. If your breathing starts to improve, increase your intensity; if you feel more congested, ease up.	Don't exercise while taking over-the-counter antihistamines, which can speed your heart rate.
Flu	If you're experiencing symptoms below the neck, such as a cough, muscle aches, or phlegm in your chest, don't exercise—period.	Once you feel better, begin at 40 percent of your normal intensity and time; increase both by 10 percent daily.	Exercising with a fever could harm your heart and your immune system. Give your body the rest it needs.
Hangover	Alcohol and exercise can both cause blood vessels to enlarge. "Combining the two can make your blood pressure fall to a low level," says Dr. Weinberg.	Stick with a less intense activity, such as stretching or yoga.	Alcohol is dehydrating, so drink at least 32 ounces of water prior to your workout and an additional 8 ounces every 15 minutes during the workout.
Jet lag	Changing time zones means scrambling your body's internal clock, which can leave you feeling sluggish and sleepy. Exercise can help reset that clock.	Give your body at least a day to adjust. When you're ready, begin exercising at about half your normal intensity.	Grogginess usually causes a loss of coordination. Choose exercises that require less balance, such as seated movements instead of standing exercises.

tap into that same spirit by giving yourself a little goal to shoot for, says Brick. "Even something as simple as planning to walk in a 5-K for charity can be all the motivation you need to get out there and keep going."

Build yourself up. The fear of failure can be a huge barrier to your success in a fitness program. It's something we all face, no matter how old or young or confident we are, says exercise physiologist Robert Brosmer, vice president of health and wellness at the Central Florida YMCA in Orlando and coauthor of *Health and High Performance*.

"Fear of failing is especially daunting in the beginning, when maybe you don't feel as sure of your abilities as you'd like," he says. "A good way to beat down that fear is to build up your confidence. Make a list of all the difficult tasks in your life you've accomplished: raising children, buying a home, getting a degree, and so on. Then, when you start to feel your confidence flagging, say to yourself, 'If I could accomplish those things, I'm sure I can accomplish this.'"

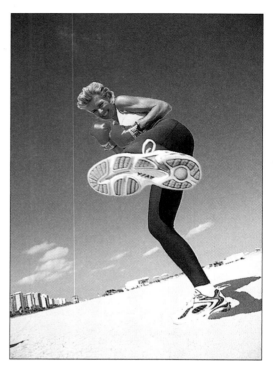

A good way to beat down the fear of failing is to list the difficult tasks **you've accomplished in your life**.

Health Problems? Shape Up the Right Way

People who have a chronic health problem need a specially tailored exercise program. Here's how to choose the right exercises and, with your doctor's help, take the right precautions if you have arthritis, diabetes, or hypertension. The following tips are particularly important.

• Warm up first, to boost circulation, prevent a sudden rise in blood pressure, and loosen stiff muscles and joints.

• Avoid high-impact exercise, which can raise blood pressure excessively, break fragile blood vessels, and injure arthritic joints and nerve-damaged feet.

• Exercise indoors when it's cold outside. Cold weather stiffens the joints, increases blood pressure, and further numbs nerve-impaired feet.

• Cool down after working out. By walking slowly and then stretching, you will prevent a dangerous drop in blood pressure and maintain joint mobility.

Here are additional guidelines specific to each ailment.

Arthritis

People with arthritis, particularly rheumatoid arthritis, should stretch the affected joints every day, even when those joints are inflamed. It's also important to strengthen the joints.

• Start with isometric exercises: Tense the muscles without moving the joint and without holding your breath.

• If possible, progress to isotonics such as weight lifting.

• When you have little or no pain or inflammation, work on improving your stamina by doing low-impact aerobic exercises such as walking, cycling, swimming, or dancing.

• Two particularly safe and effective workouts are calisthenics in a heated pool and tai chi, a relaxing exercise that features slow, sweeping movements.

Diabetes

Aerobic exercise can help control diabetes directly, by improving your body's use of sugar, as well as indirectly, by facilitating weight loss. Exercise is safest and most effective for people with type 2 diabetes, the most common form of the disease. But certain precautions are still essential.

• Be sure your blood sugar level is reasonably well-controlled before you start an exercise program.

• Before and after workouts that put stress on your feet, check them for blisters, breaks in the skin, redness, or swelling.

• Check your blood sugar level before and after exercising.

• Don't lift heavy weights. Straining raises your blood pressure and can damage blood vessels.

Hypertension

Regular aerobic exercise produces temporary and sometimes lasting reductions in blood pressure.

• Moderately intense exercise (60 to 70 percent of your maximum heart rate) lowers blood pressure at least as effectively as more intense exercise does. (For a rough estimate of your maximum heart rate, subtract your age from 220.)

• Avoid strenuous exertion, which can push your blood pressure to a dangerously high level.

Chapter 10

The No-Exercise Way to Burn Fat

It's easy. It's fun. And it doesn't take a huge time commitment.

Until recently, it seemed that the only way to solve the burn-more-calories part of the weight-loss equation was to sweat it out at the gym for an hour or so several times a week. Not so. Research shows that moderate activity can burn fat just as efficiently as a structured exercise program.

In a groundbreaking study from Johns Hopkins University in Baltimore, a group of overweight women who simply started walking, gardening, or generally being more active about 30 minutes a day lost as much weight—about 18 pounds—as a similar group who did step aerobics three times a week.

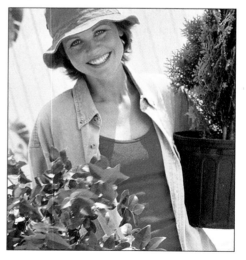

Even better, a year later, the women doing the less rigorous activities regained less than half a pound, on average. The women on the exercise program gained back 3½ pounds.

That's right. You don't have to join a gym, strap on a heart rate monitor, or any of the other expensive equipment that so-called fitness gurus have been trying to get you to buy for the last 20 years.

All you have to do is have some fun.

Make Fitness Last, Make It Fun

It's hard to believe that fitness is so simple after years of hearing (and feeling!) how hard it was. "No pain, no gain" was the credo we were taught to live by.

And if we didn't "work out" for at least 20 minutes at our "target heart rate" at least 3 days a week, we were told that we weren't doing any good. No wonder so many folks quit!

Today fitness experts know better, says exercise physiologist Robert Brosmer, vice president of health and wellness at the Central Florida YMCA in Orlando and coauthor of *Health and High Performance.*

"In the beginning, fitness experts weren't being taken seriously, so they responded by making exercise a very serious business," Brosmer says. "And while we were running around talking about target heart rates, a lot of people quit exercising. Now we know what really matters is getting off the couch and getting a little active, even if it's just for 10 minutes at lunch and 10 minutes in the evening on a regular basis."

The best part is that you can get fit by doing things you love, says Paul Konstanty, clinical supervisor and exercise therapist at the University of California OrthoMed Spine and Joint Conditioning Center in San Diego.

Outsmart Your Fat Gene

You just can't avoid some family traits. But new research suggests that your activity level can override a genetic tendency to gain weight.

When scientists compared nearly 350 middle-age female twins, they discovered that the twin who was more active was slimmer than her sister, despite having the same genetic risk for being overweight.

Although activity of any kind helped, the researchers found that the more the women moved, the better their chances were of getting and staying trim, says study author Katherine Samaras, M.D., of St. Vincent's Clinic in Sydney, Australia.

To really blast fat, try hiking, biking, stairclimbing, or raking leaves—anything that'll make you break a sweat.

Every Step Counts

Instead of thinking of exercise as pain and sweat, think of it as your body in motion—any kind of motion. Or to put it another way: The more you move your arms and legs, the more calories you burn. The more you sit or lie still, the fewer calories you burn.

The problem is, we're doing too much sitting and too little moving. Blame our harried schedules or the conveniences of modern technology. With the click of a switch, we can open a garage door, change the channel on the TV, or go shopping all over the globe. All in all, fewer than one in four of us gets the 30 minutes of daily activity recommended by health experts. That's a lot of unspent calories.

According to a study from the United Kingdom, people there burn about 800 calories less per day than they did in 1970, mostly because of automation and labor-saving devices. It's the same story on this side of the Atlantic.

"Physical activity has been pushed out of our lives," says Miriam Nelson, Ph.D., associate chief of the Human Physiology Laboratory at the Jean Mayer USDA Human Nutrition Research Center on Aging at Tufts University in Boston and author of *Strong Women Stay Slim*. "It is no longer a part of our social fabric. This means we have to choose ways to work activity back into our lives. We have to consciously get up more, walk more, take the stairs more. Whenever possible, we need to seek out activity."

Most moderate-intensity activities, such as walking briskly, raking leaves, mowing the lawn with a push mower, or vacuuming, will burn 150 calories in about 30 minutes. So instead of just counting calories, also add up your minutes of activity each day. To lose weight and keep it off, you actually need about 60 minutes of activity a day, according to the latest research.

It doesn't make any difference if you do it all at once or break it up into smaller chunks of time. "Everything counts," says Barbara Moore, Ph.D., president of Shape Up America!, a national physical fitness coalition based in Washington, D.C.

Step up the intensity. Michelle L. Edwards, a health educator at the Cooper Insti-

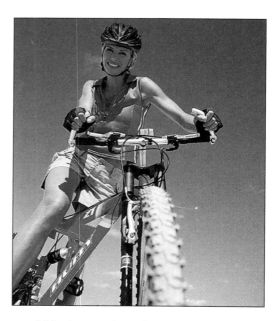

We have to choose ways to work activity back into our lives. Whenever possible, **we need to seek out activity**.

tute for Aerobics Research in Dallas and a certified personal trainer, advises her clients to start by simply increasing the intensity of any physical activity that they're already doing. That can mean taking the stairs a little faster, choosing parking spots at the far end of the lot, or making wider arm circles when wiping the kitchen counter. The idea is to put a little more effort into every activity in order to burn more calories.

Keep a diary. For the next few days, clock yourself every time you walk, clean, garden, climb a flight of stairs, or perform any other activity that involves moving the muscles in your arms and legs. At the end of the day, add up your active time. This helps to create a vivid picture of how the minutes add up, explains Edwards. Once you do this, you'll probably find yourself thinking of all kinds of ways to add a few more minutes here and there throughout the day.

One of the keys to becoming more active is learning to identify opportunities in your day and taking advantage of them. "Five minutes here; 10 minutes there. It all adds up," notes Edwards.

It also helps to do the reverse—record how much time you spend sitting each day. Figure out ways to gradually reduce that amount.

Get a pedometer. If you want to get a clearer picture of the amount of physical activity you are doing in a day, record how many steps you take on an average day and then find ways to add more. Studies show that people who are active for 30 minutes each day accumulate about 10,000 steps, while the average person who works in an office typically takes about

Burning Calories

If you are a 150-pound woman, how long does it take to burn 150 more calories a day? That depends on what you do. (If you weigh more, it may take less intensity to burn the same amount of calories.)

- Ironing for 59 minutes
- Cooking for 48 minutes
- Washing and waxing a car for 45 to 60 minutes
- Playing volleyball for 45 minutes
- Strolling through the mall for 44 minutes
- Grocery shopping for 36 minutes
- Doing yoga for 36 minutes
- Vacuuming for 34 minutes
- Playing horseshoes for 33 minutes
- Gardening for 30 to 45 minutes
- Bicycling at a leisurely pace for 5 miles in 30 minutes
- Brisk walking for 30 minutes
- Dancing fast for 30 minutes
- Pushing a stroller for 30 minutes
- Raking leaves for 30 minutes

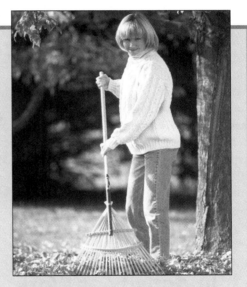

- Mowing the lawn with a power push mower for 29 minutes
- Inline skating at a leisurely pace for 26 minutes
- Stacking firewood for 25 minutes
- Bowling for 23 minutes
- Scrubbing floors for 20 minutes
- Swimming for 19 minutes
- Climbing stairs for 15 minutes
- Shoveling snow for 15 minutes

2,000 to 4,000 steps a day. "A pedometer can be a very motivational tool, a way to self-monitor," says Edwards. "And we know from experience that people who self-monitor are more likely to reach their activity goals than people who do not."

Be prepared. Keep walking shoes in your car or desk so that you can walk whenever you have a few minutes, suggest Edwards.

Schedule it. We tend to keep our appointments, so make an appointment to exercise. You can start by scheduling exercise in the morning instead of later in the day, suggests Denise Bruner, M.D., president of the American Society of Bariatric Physicians and a physician practicing in Arlington, Virginia. "Women seem to be more successful in general if they put activity on the front end of the day versus the end of the day, when either work-related issues or home issues can end up taking precedence over exercise time," she says.

Working In Activity at Work

A hundred years ago, the average woman burned about 50 percent more calories a day. There was no need to worry about making sure you moved your body enough. Movement was built into each and every day.

"Basically, at the turn of the 20th century, something like 85 percent of our workforce worked in agricultural-related jobs," says Dr. Moore. "These jobs were very physically demanding. In today's information-based society, so

---

1-MINUTE FAT BURNER

Fidget. You can burn up to 700 calories a day!

---

much of the work we do requires sitting and only sitting."

Besides sleeping, a lot of us spend the biggest chunk of our time at work. If you can work in three 10-minute walks over the course of your day, you'll burn an extra 150 calories. In a year, that adds up to more than 10 pounds of fat-burning calories. Here's how you can work in a workout.

Park on the outskirts. As in most cities, parking is scarce in Boston. Dr. Nelson ends up parking about eight blocks from her office each day. But instead of taking the university-provided shuttle, she walks the rest of the way. "I get an 8-minute walk every morning and afternoon. Then I add in a little bit here and there, and before you know it, I've burned a fair number of calories," she says.

Change your bus stop. If you use public transportation, you probably already do a fair amount of walking. If you want to add a few more steps to your day, Dr. Moore recommends getting off your mode of transit a few stops early.

Take advantage of the speakerphone. Walk around or do stretches while you're on the phone, says Dr. Moore. Standing burns about 30 percent more calories than sitting.

Seek out the stairs instead of the elevator. "Buildings are designed so that the elevator is prominent and the stairs are not," says Dr. Moore. Stairways are tucked away in the far corners of the building and may not seem accessible. Seek them out. "Every opportunity should be seized to take a few steps." If you work in a high-rise, get off the elevator a few floors early and take the stairs the rest of the way. Add more floors as you build stamina.

Schedule a mobile meeting. Instead of sitting in a conference room and meeting over a cup of coffee, schedule a walking meeting, suggests Edwards.

Take the long way around. Whenever you're walking somewhere, take the long route, whether you're headed to the mail room or the conference room, says Dr. Nelson. Remember, every extra minute of walking burns about 5 calories.

Use the restroom on another floor. Or, if you work in a one-story building, use the restroom farthest away from your desk, suggests Dr. Moore.

Set an activity timer. Program your computer or watch to remind you to take a brief walk, says Bess H. Marcus, Ph.D., associate professor of psychiatry and human behavior at the Brown University Center for Behavioral and Preventive Medicine in Providence, Rhode Island. Set your watch to go off each hour to re-

HealthPoint

Boost Your Brainpower in Just 3 Days

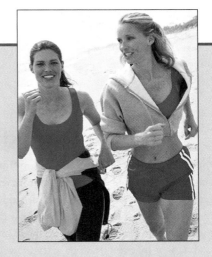

Start walking now—even if you're over 60 and never exercised a day in your life—and you can look forward to being more quick-witted in your golden years.

Researchers split 124 sedentary adults ages 60 to 75 into two groups: One group walked briskly 3 days a week (progressing from 15 to 45 minutes); the other group did stretching and toning exercises for 1 hour, three times a week. After 6 months, the walkers significantly improved their scores on computer tasks, while the calisthenics group had no improvements.

The part of the brain responsible for managing multiple tasks, ignoring distractions, and calling on memory tends to decline first, explains study author Arthur Kramer, Ph.D., professor of psychology at the University of Illinois at Urbana–Champaign. But walking increases oxygen flow to the brain and appears to slow these declines.

"Walking just 3 days a week translates into a 15 percent boost in mental functioning, which is substantial for such a small investment in time," says Dr. Kramer. It can make the difference between easily juggling preparations for a four-course meal and burning dinner.

mind you to take a 5-minute walk. At the end of the workday, you could easily accumulate 30 to 40 minutes of activity.

Order out. Build activity into your lunch hour. Instead of using the entire hour or half-hour to eat, save at least 10 minutes for a brisk walk. Or, you could try ordering your lunch from a restaurant that's six blocks away instead of one that's right around the corner, and then walk to get it, says Dr. Nelson.

Never take the escalator down. No, you don't burn as many calories walking down the steps as you do going up, but it's still an opportunity to move those muscles, says Dr. Moore. To boost your burn, swing your arms as you're walking down the stairs or downhill.

Activate Your Life Everyday

Our harried home lives often feel anything but inactive. We're constantly on the go from the moment our feet hit the floor in the morning until the last chore is done at night. Who has time to squeeze one more thing onto their to-do list? The good news is that you don't have to do more; you just need to do it differently. You can find hidden opportunities for exercise simply by changing your approach to everyday chores and errands.

Don't let things pile up when you pick up. Eliminate using the bottom stairs as a holding area for stuff that needs to go on another floor, says Dr. Moore. Walk up and down the stairs every time you come across something that needs to be put away.

Walk and talk. Don't settle into your favorite chair for a good, long tête-à-tête when your best friend calls. Take advantage of the mobility you get using the cordless phone. Walk around, put away odds and ends, or go up and down the stairs while you talk.

Be an active captive. "Think if there is some way for you to get more activity while you're a captive at your child's activities," says Dr. Marcus. Walk around the soccer field while watching the game. Take a walk around the block during the half-hour piano lesson.

Get lean while you clean. We're spending about 18 hours a week doing housework—half the time our mothers spent. "I always recommend that people do housework to boost their activity levels," says Dr. Moore. We're not suggesting you step back into the days of domestic drudgery, but when you do clean, use large, exaggerated movements to burn more calories.

Do your own yard work. Don't hire a neighborhood kid. If you do an hour of yard work a week, you'll burn about 300 extra calories. But don't use a power mower. "If you do, you won't burn 300 calories of your fat. You'll burn gasoline instead," says Dr. Moore.

Tote more groceries. It seems much more efficient to try and lug all the groceries into the house in one trip. But you can burn more calories if you make multiple trips and bring the bags in one at a time, says Dr. Moore.

Go back to basics. Find places in your day where you can do a task in a more manual way, says Dr. Nelson. Get out the hose and wash your car yourself instead of taking it to the car wash. Lose your remote control and get up off the couch to switch channels. Walk to the store for a gallon of milk.

Chapter 11

Walk Off Weight Your Way

It's a busy woman's easiest exercise.

It's as simple as putting one foot in front of another. But if you do it every day, you can lose weight, increase your energy, lower your risk of chronic disease, boost your brainpower, calm your nerves, improve your mood, and live longer. Not a bad list of advantages for something that you learned how to do before you could talk.

Walking is something we can—and should—do every day. Every extra step we take goes a long way toward improving our health. In a study of almost 16,000 twins, Finnish researchers found that those who took about six ½-hour walks a month were 30 percent less likely to die during the study than their more sedentary siblings.

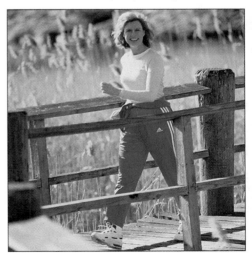

"There is no better exercise than walking," says John Yetter, M.D., medical director at SSM Rehab

Sports Medicine in St. Louis. "It makes you feel younger, more fit, and energized. If I can get people out walking about 20 minutes 3 or 4 days a week, I know they'll be hooked."

Feel-Good Benefits

Walk regularly, and your body will burn more calories and more fat all day long because you've revved up your metabolism. You'll also help tone your abdominals, hips, thighs, and buttocks.

"Instead of buying some 'miracle' weight-loss gimmick, all you really need to do is walk," says James Rippe, M.D., associate professor at Tufts University School of Medicine in Boston, director of the Center of Clinical and Lifestyle Research in Shrewsbury, Massachusetts, and author of *Fit Over Forty*.

The benefits of walking are so dramatic that it's worth taking a look at them one by one.

A youthful waistline. "We always point the finger at fast food when we talk about the overweight problem in this country, but it has more to do with our increasingly inactive lifestyles," says Dr. Rippe. "Something as simple as walking can help prevent the weight gain we associate with middle age."

Don't think walking can burn enough calories to whittle your waistline? Consider this: Brisk walking—about 4½ miles an hour—actually burns more calories than running at the same pace, according to a study from Washington University in St. Louis.

A younger heart. Probably the best benefit of regular walking is a stronger, healthier heart. The Centers for Disease Control and Prevention reports that walking just 3 hours a week at an easy pace can cut your risk for heart attack and stroke by almost a third. The same 3 hours, when you walk a little faster, can cut these risks in half.

"It doesn't matter how old you are; walking can improve your cardiovascular fitness, control blood pressure, lower cholesterol, and improve the tone of your arteries," says Dr. Rippe. "All of those things not only help you live longer, but help you look and feel healthier and younger."

Healthy blood sugar. A regular walking program is one of the best strategies for easing symptoms of diabetes as well as preventing it in the first place, says Dr. Rippe. In a study of more than 1,400 men and women, researchers at the University of South Carolina, Columbia, found that taking a daily walk significantly improved how well the body used insulin to regulate blood sugar.

Sound sleep. When we're young and without worry, we generally sleep straight through the night (and sometimes well into the morning!) without much trouble. As we get older, the responsibilities that come with aging can rob us of this restful luxury. Regular walking can give it back, says Dr. Yetter. Researchers at the University of Arizona have found that regular

Walking burns **100 calories per mile** if you weigh 150 pounds.

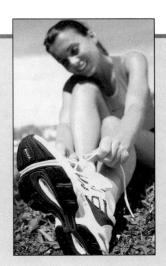

The Right Shoe

The top priority for all walkers is good shoes. Here is what Bonnie Stein, a nationally known racewalking instructor and coach in Redington Shores, Florida, recommends that you look for when you shop for shoes.

Flexibility. The shoe should bend where your foot bends—at the ball of your foot, not in the middle of the shoe.

An ample toebox. When you walk, you bend and push off with your toes. There should be a thumb's width from the end of your longest toe to the front end of the shoe, says Stein. If the toebox isn't big enough, your toes will be tingling 20 minutes into your walk.

Light, thin materials. Look for walking shoes that are lightweight, with a thin heel and a flexible sole. Running and walking shoes with soles that are extremely thick and cushioned are not good for walking. Also stay away from aerobics, tennis, and basketball shoes, Stein says. Cross-trainers are too stiff and inflexible for walking and don't offer the proper support.

walking lowers the risk for all kinds of sleep problems, including fitful and interrupted sleep.

Fewer aches and pains. At least 80 percent of people in this country will be waylaid with back pain at some point. And let's face it, the more years we live, the better the chances our backs will let us down. But instead of resting on your behind waiting for your back to feel better, in most cases, going for walks will strengthen the back, shed some of those back-straining pounds, and generally make you feel better, says Dr. Yetter. Don't forget to stretch before going for a walk—stretching adds flexibility to the back.

Stress relief. Walking makes you feel better. If you want proof, just ask the women

who take walking classes from nationally known racewalking instructor and coach Bonnie Stein in Redington Shores, Florida. A study of 25 women in one of Stein's walking classes showed that 48 percent of them showed signs of stress, and almost half had been in therapy for depression. By the end of the 8-week program, only 32 percent of the women showed signs of stress.

Walking Workouts

Beginners should aim for a level of exertion equivalent to a 6 or 7 on a scale of 1 to 10, advises Stein. You should be able to carry on a conversation without being short of breath.

Another way to measure exertion is to monitor your heart rate. To calculate your target heart rate, subtract your age from 220, then multiply by the level of exertion at which you want to exercise (60 percent of your maximum is good for beginners). For example, if you are 50 years old and want to start out at 60 percent exertion, the math would work like this: $220 - 50 = 170$; $170 \times 0.60 = 102$.

Thus, your heart rate should be 102 beats per minute when you walk. As you develop endurance and lose weight, increase your walking time and the intensity by recalculating your target heart rate at a higher percentage or by aiming for an exertion level of 7 or 8.

Beginner: 20 minutes 6 or 7 days a week for 2 weeks

Intermediate: 25 minutes 6 or 7 days a week; increase walking time in 10-percent increments each week until you reach 40 minutes

Experienced: Continue to increase walking time by 10 percent until you reach 45 to 60 minutes 6 or 7 days a week. If you don't need to lose body fat, you can walk 20 to 30 minutes 3 days a week to stay fit.

Customize Your Walking Technique

You took your first steps somewhere around your first year of life and have been striding around

---

1-MINUTE FAT BURNER

Sip green tea before you walk. The caffeine frees fatty acids so that you burn fat more easily. And the polyphenols (antioxidant compounds) in green tea appear to work with caffeine to increase calorie burn.

---

ever since. That's the beauty of walking. You don't need to learn a thing. You can just step out your door and go. The other great thing about walking is that you can always pick up new tips and techniques to make this simple exercise even better, notes Stein.

"Any kind of walking can be good for you," Stein says. "But if you want to really lose weight and feel fitter and younger, you have to adjust your technique and pick up the pace a little bit."

Take short, quick steps instead of long strides. Short steps will work your glute muscles (in your buttocks) as you log miles, says Kate Larsen, a walking instructor and certified group fitness instructor in Minneapolis.

Rock on your feet. You'll burn more calories if you put your whole body into your stride, says Stein. "Concentrate on pushing off. Think about rolling from your heel, through the outside of your foot, to the ball of your toes, and then pushing off from the toes." Your front stride will be short and quick, rather than long and leisurely.

Swing your arms. Normal walking is great for strengthening your legs. But if you want to give your upper body a more youthful tone, you have to get your arms involved, says Stein. "Swinging your arms can improve the effectiveness of your walking 100 percent. You'll go faster and get some firming and toning of the upper arms," she explains.

Start by bending your arms at about a 90-degree angle. Hold your arms in close enough to your body so your thumb brushes just under your waistband as your arms move forward and back. Close your fists loosely and bring them up just about to your sternum on the upswing. Swing them slightly behind the side seam of your shorts on the downswing. "Concentrate on streamlining your body like a rocket by keeping your elbows pulled in and your arms swinging smoothly and rhythmically," Stein says.

Squeeze your glutes. Imagine squeezing and lifting your glutes up and back, as if you were holding a $50 bill between them. This will strengthen and tone your glute muscles. Developing the ability to maintain this deep contraction throughout your walk will take a while.

"Zip up" your abs. During your walk, imagine that you're zipping up a tight pair of jeans. Stand tall and pull your abdominal muscles up and in. You can practice this even when you're not walking. This will also strengthen your lower-back muscles.

The Quickest Way to Start a Walking Habit

Finding time to exercise just got easier. You can squeeze in your walks—with all their benefits—in less time than ever.

When researchers put 32 sedentary adults on one of three brisk walking programs (30 minutes all at one time; three 10-minute sessions throughout the day; or any combination of at least 5-minute sessions, totaling 30 minutes per day), those who walked as little as 5 minutes at a time improved their cardiovascular fitness and decreased blood pressure as much as the others—and they had an easier time making it a habit.

"Five-minute bouts are easier to fit into busy schedules, so you're more likely to do it and to stick with it," says study author Karen Coleman, Ph.D., assistant professor of health psychology at the University of Texas at El Paso. When all of the groups increased their walking from 3 to 6 days a week, the 5-minute walkers effortlessly met the challenge, while walkers in the other groups had more difficulty finding time.

Next time you're waiting for muffins in the oven, or your hairdresser is running late, use the opportunity to sneak in a walk, and you'll rack up extra miles effortlessly. For best results, walk at a brisk pace, as though you're in a hurry to get somewhere.

Stand tall. An upright posture makes your walking more efficient by opening up your chest, allowing your lungs to expand fully. Imagine that there's a string attached to the top of your head, and that it's pulling you slightly skyward with every stride. Keep your eyes up and focused about 12 to 20 feet ahead of you. This will keep your neck aligned properly.

Take the talk test. Walking is supposed to be invigorating and fun. You shouldn't be gasping for air, but your body shouldn't be bored, either. "On a scale of 1 to 10, with 1 being lying in bed and 10 being all-out exertion, I tell people to aim for about a 7," Stein says.

One way to tell if you're hitting the right stride is to do the "talk test," she advises. "When you're walking at a 7, you should be breathing harder than normal, but you should still be able to carry on a simple conversation."

Walk every day. To get the best results, you really should try to walk every day, says Stein. "If you aim to do it every day, you'll probably get 5 or 6 days in every week. If you shoot for fewer, you'll walk fewer."

Take a 10-minute walking break. Obviously, the longer you walk, the fitter you'll get. But in a busy world, it's not always possible to break away for a half-hour at a time. Don't sweat it. Just take a 10-minute walk around the block, says Marie H. Murphy, Ph.D., exercise physiologist at the University of Ulster at Jordanstown, Northern Ireland. British researchers have found that short bouts of brisk walking—say three 10-minute walks—yield similar fat-burning benefits as walking the same amount all at once.

"We've found that taking 10-minute walks might even be better in the long run," says Dr. Murphy, who coauthored the study. "If you're set

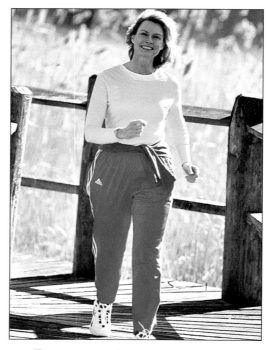

For more than 75 percent of people in the National Weight Control Registry who have successfully lost weight—and kept it off— **walking is the answer**.

on the idea of walking 30 minutes a day, and then you miss a session, you've missed a full 30 minutes that week. If you miss one 10-minute session, you've missed much less."

Make It Fun!

Once you've started walking regularly, there are literally dozens of ways to keep it fresh and maximally effective. Here are some ideas to get you started.

Take a hike. Hiking can be described as adventurous walking where the sidewalk ends. It's a wonderful way to enjoy the benefits of walking to the fullest and explore the great outdoors, says Michelle L. Edwards, a health educator at the Cooper Institute for Aerobics Research in Dallas and a certified personal trainer. "There are hiking clubs in almost every community. You can join them on day hikes along the most beautiful trails in your area," she says. Hiking also burns tons of calories: about 400 an hour for a 150-pound person moving at a leisurely pace. Visit the American Hiking Society's Web site at www.americanhiking.org for a list of hiking clubs in your area.

Go to the mall. Not a big fan of the outdoors? Many shopping malls open their doors (but not their stores) early in the morning so people can come in and walk, says Edwards. "That way, you can lighten your waistline without lightening your wallet!"

Try pole-walking. A fun way to add some zip to your step and burn almost a quarter more calories is to walk with trekking poles, says Edwards. These are rubber-tipped ski poles designed for walking. Studies have found that the effort it takes to swing the poles while you walk burns more calories and increases your heart rate by about 15 percent.

Tune into tunes. It's not the best idea to wear headphones when you're walking outdoors because it's too hard to hear what's going on around you. But inside, when you're mall-walking or walking on a treadmill, music can make the time fly. "People work out longer and at a higher intensity while listening to music, even when they don't mean to," Edwards says.

Make walking feel like play. When you were a kid, you didn't go out and play in order to think about your homework. You did it to stretch your body, air out your mind, and have some fun. Treat walking the same way, says Dr. Yetter. "Treat it as a break from the daily grind. Make it as fun as possible by exploring new neighborhoods and parks. Admire the way people decorate their yards. Watch birds. Clear your mind and relax."

Chapter 12

Trade Fat for Muscle in 10 Minutes a Day

Burn more fat automatically without eating less or exercising more!

Forget everything you've heard about muscle and bulk: Muscle tissue is what keeps you thin. Each pound of lean muscle tissue in your body burns about 50 calories a day, even when you're not doing anything more than sitting around. Each pound of fat tissue burns only 2 calories.

This is one of the reasons you could eat more when you were younger and not gain weight. Pound for pound, you naturally had more calorie-burning muscle tissue. The problem is, when women reach their forties, they start losing small amounts of muscle and replacing it with fat. After age 40, you naturally lose about ½ pound of muscle every year.

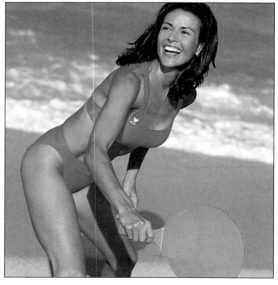

Why Your Size Matters

Finding moves that match your height could bring your workout to new levels.

You exercise to improve your body—but if you're fairly short or tall, your body may be holding you back. "Being above or below average height can put you at a biomechanical disadvantage when you exercise," says Heather Dillinger, a certification specialist for the Aerobic and Fitness Association of America. "Some exercises require movements that compromise benefits or cause injury." Try these recommendations.

If You're 5'10" or Above

Skip: Squats. Tall women absorb more pressure in the lower back trying to keep the spine straight during squats.

Try: Dumbbell lunges. This move won't put pressure on the spine. Stand with your feet hip-width apart and hold a light dumbbell in each hand. Step forward as far as you can with your right foot, bending your right knee (keep your knee directly above your ankle). Return to the starting position; repeat with your left leg.

If You're 5'2" or Below

Skip: Leg-curl machines. Shorter women's hips bend before the curve in the bench, forcing them to shimmy farther back on the machine, which stresses the back.

Try: Straight-leg dumbbell dead lifts. This exercise targets the hamstrings effectively, but it's easier on your lower back. Stand with your feet shoulder-width apart. Let your arms hang down, holding 5- to 10-pound weights in front of your thighs. With your back flat and your abs contracted, flex forward at the hip; lower weights to the floor. Keeping your back straight, use your leg and butt muscles to rise again.

Skip: Chest-press machines. Handles on these machines tend to be spaced too far apart for shorter women to grasp, which can cause elbow and shoulder strain.

Try: Dumbbell press. Without the locked-grip position, you can keep your hands directly in line with your elbows. For your chest, lie on a bench with your knees bent, feet flat on the bench, and a weight in each hand. With palms facing forward, push the weights upward until your arms are extended above your chest, keeping your elbows bent. Lower the weights along the sides of your chest and repeat.

Some women lose up to 1 pound a year once they hit menopause. At that rate, you could be down 15 pounds of muscle and burning 600 fewer calories a day by the time you are well into menopause.

Luckily, it doesn't have to be that way.

Muscle Makes You Trim and Shapely

Strength training will not only give you your old body back, it will give you a better body back. Aerobic activity can burn calories and fat, but only strength training will tone you, give you a great shape, and rev up your metabolism.

Exercise physiologists used to emphasize aerobics as the best way to get in shape. But we're now finding that strength training is at least as effective for total health and fitness, says exercise physiologist Robert Brosmer, vice president of health and wellness at the Central Florida YMCA in Orlando and coauthor of *Health and High Performance*. "Only strength training and sensible nutritional habits really change the way you look."

Though men have been taking advantage of the toning effects of weight lifting for years, women are just starting to discover that strength training is just what they've been looking for to fight the effects of age and gravity—especially in their curves!

"Women are very specific about the body parts they want to make better," says Majid Ali, a certified fitness instructor in Los Angeles. "They want to firm their butts and lift their breasts and stop places from jiggling. Though aerobic exercise can certainly help you lose weight all over, the best way to hit these spots is to build those muscles."

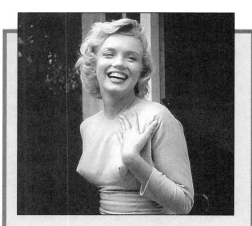

HOLLYWOOD HEALTH

Bombshell with Dumbbells

Most people don't know that Marilyn Monroe lifted weights. That's right: That American icon of femininity, beauty, and glamour hoisted dumbbells regularly. Obviously, she didn't want bigger muscles or to look more masculine. She just knew what millions of women are discovering today— that building muscle is among the best ways to keep a young, trim figure.

Muscle Makes You Young

Building muscle does more than give you a younger-looking body. It also gives you a younger-feeling body.

"People can't believe how much physical improvement they notice once they start resistance training," says Laura Senft, a physical therapist at Kessler Institute for Rehabilitation in West Orange, New Jersey. "They can do everything better, from climbing stairs to playing with their kids. They have more energy. And because they're reducing body fat, building bone, and increasing muscle, they're a whole lot healthier."

Here are some of the ways that weight lifting helps make your body young.

It revs your metabolism. In a Tufts University study, after just 12 weeks, people who increased their muscle mass by 3 pounds could eat 15 percent more calories—that's 225 calories if you normally eat a 1,500-calorie diet—without gaining an ounce. "And on average, they still lost 4 pounds of fat," says Wayne Westcott, Ph.D., fitness research director at the South Shore YMCA in Quincy, Massachusetts.

Strength training gives you more lean muscle tissue, which burns tons of calories every day. It also gives your metabolism an extra calorie-burning boost for about 30 minutes after you're done working out. In fact, your body continues to burn more calories after a half-hour of strength training than it does after a half-hour of jogging.

It builds younger bones. All women are at risk for osteoporosis. As our bones age, they lose calcium and other minerals. This makes them more porous and likely to break. It's also what causes some women to shrink as they age as a result of vertebrae compressing.

Strength training is the best strategy for keeping your bones strong. "Working out with some weights twice a week is all it takes to increase bone mass in your arms and legs, where women are most likely to get weak," says Senft.

It improves self-confidence. "Resistance training is great for building self-esteem," says John Yetter, M.D., medical director at SSM Rehab Sports Medicine in St. Louis. "You can see yourself getting stronger—not just when it comes to lifting weights, but in everyday life. You can climb stairs more easily. You can open jars and pick up heavy household objects. It gives you little morale boosts all day long."

It gives you better balance. When we're young and running around all the time, balance isn't much of a problem. As we get a little older and more sedentary, however, our brain-to-muscle connections can get weak from disuse. Strength training can prevent that from happening. In a study of men and women in their late seventies, researchers found that those who strength-trained three times a week for 16 weeks were able to improve their balance by almost 70 percent.

It strengthens joints. When it comes to aches, pains, and injuries, your body's weakest links are its joints. Strength training helps keep joints strong and pain-free. "It's important to strengthen your muscles, ligaments, and tendons because they're what you rely on to move through this life," says Dr. Yetter. "You won't walk, play, or work very well if your joints or muscles are weak."

You can see yourself getting stronger—
not just when it comes to lifting weights, but in everyday life.

‖ Limber Up!

Of all the exercises you can do to strengthen muscles, look fit, and feel younger, stretching is by far the quickest and easiest. Unfortunately, it's also the most overlooked, and that's a serious mistake.

Some loss of flexibility is natural as we age, but the main cause of stiffness is simply a lack of movement, says Majid Ali, certified fitness instructor in Los Angeles. "Our muscles become more calcified with disuse, so they're less pliable and not as responsive when we do try to move them," he explains.

HealthPoint

Lose Fat, Not Bone

If you're dieting, you may be losing more than body fat. In a University of Pittsburgh study, women who lost an average of 7 pounds also lost significant bone mineral density in the process.

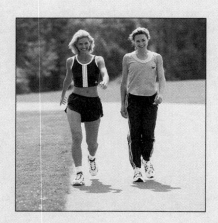

This isn't to say that you should forget about losing those excess pounds. "We definitely want to encourage people to lose excess weight, because the number one killer of women is cardiovascular disease, and extra pounds increase risk of heart disease," says university researcher Loran M. Salamone, Ph.D.

The solution? Choose weight-loss tactics that build bone, she says. Here's how.

Get 3 to 4 hours of weight-bearing aerobic exercise weekly. Weight-bearing exercise, such as walking, running, and aerobic dancing, burns calories while strengthening bone.

Add resistance training two or three times a week. Resistance training (preferably with free weights) is tops for building muscle, and is more likely to build or maintain bone mass, says Janet Shaw, Ph.D., assistant professor of exercise and sport science at the University of Utah in Salt Lake City.

Include calcium-fortified orange juice and fat-free and low-fat milk, cheese, and yogurt in your diet. You'll get lots of bone-building calcium and other nutrients for relatively few calories. If you're premenopausal, shoot for 1,000 milligrams of calcium a day from food and supplements. Take in 1,500 milligrams daily if you're past menopause.

Making matters worse is our sit-down society. Sitting all day in cars, at desks, at computers, and in front of the TV not only makes us overweight, it shortens our hip flexor muscles and rounds our shoulders so we become stiff and hunched over.

Thankfully, we can reverse this simply by stretching, says Joy Lynn Freeman, D.C., a chiropractor and stretching instructor in Prescott, Arizona, and author of *Express Yourself.* "Stretching makes your body more beautiful," she says. "You stand taller, appear slimmer, and move more freely when you stretch regularly. The more limber you are, the younger you feel. It's like a youth capsule."

Of course, it isn't just the inactive among us who need to stretch. It's equally important when you're active and getting in shape. Exercising your muscles without stretching can actually make them tighter. And the tighter your muscles, the more prone they are to injury. You'll be much less likely to get hurt when you stretch regularly. A bonus: Stretching muscles after a good workout will help make them stronger and also help prevent that postexercise soreness.

"A good postexercise stretch is like wringing out your muscles," says Dr. Freeman. Lactic acid and other cellular waste—the stuff that makes your muscles tender the day after a tough workout—are normal by-products of muscle use. "Stretching helps increase circulation through the muscles and flushes out those lingering waste materials," she explains.

Always warm up for at least 5 to 10 minutes before stretching. Walk around and move your muscles a bit. Stretching muscles when they're "cold" can lead to strains and tears. Hold each stretch for a slow count of 10, and repeat three times. Aim to stretch every day.

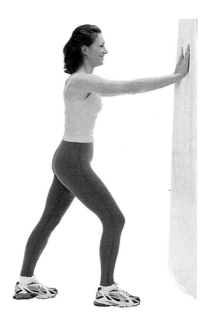

1. Calf stretch: Stand arm's length away from a wall. Place your palms flat against the wall. Extend your right leg behind you 2 to 3 feet and press your right heel to the floor. (Your left knee will bend as you extend back.) Keep both heels flat against the floor. Hold, relax, and repeat with the left leg.

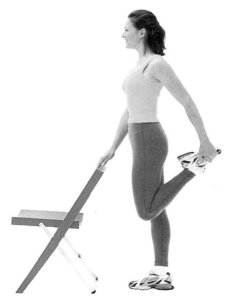

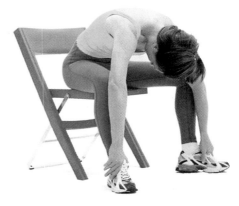

2. Quad stretch: Stand with your right hand resting on a chair or a table for support. Bend your left leg behind you. Grip the top of your left foot with your left hand and slowly pull the heel toward your rear until you feel a stretch in your quadriceps (front thigh). Be sure to keep your hips and knees aligned, and don't lock the knee of your supporting leg. Hold, relax, and repeat with your other leg.

3. Lower-back stretch: Sitting on the edge of a secure chair, bend at the waist, dropping your head and chest to your legs while reaching your hands toward your ankles. Keep your belly tight. Don't do this exercise if you have radiating leg pain.

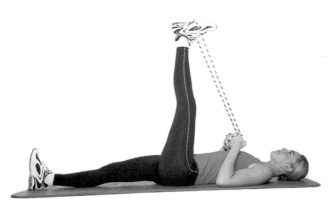

4. Hamstring stretch: Loop a towel or rope under the arch of your left foot and lie flat on your back, legs straight out on the floor. Keeping your knee straight, pull your left leg off the floor until you feel a stretch. Be sure to keep your back pressed to the floor throughout the stretch. Hold, then repeat with your other leg.

The Fat-Fighting Workout

Most people are convinced that the only way to get the benefits of strength training is to spend hours at the gym. Nothing could be further from the truth. You can get all the same benefits of a Nautilus machine—with minimal gear—right at home. It takes about 10 minutes a day, and you'll see results in just 8 weeks.

For best results, start with a weight that causes muscle fatigue after one set of 8 to 12 repetitions. "Muscles will change only when you challenge them," says Michael Hewitt, Ph.D., director of exercise physiology at Canyon Ranch Spa in Tucson. "If you can lift the weight 13 to 15 times, it probably isn't heavy enough. If you can't hoist it at least 8 times, then it's too heavy."

The key to making your body its youngest, shapeliest best is to exercise and tone all your major muscle groups. You can hit them all with 10 simple exercises. Alternate the upper- and lower-body workouts, aiming to do each two or three times a week. Allow at least one day of rest before working the same muscle group again. To maximize fat burn, include 45 minutes of aerobic exercise, such as walking, cycling, or inline skating, at least 5 days a week.

So let's get started!

For the Upper Body

1. Modified pushup: Lie facedown on the floor with your hands by your shoulders and your knees bent. Press your palms into the floor, straightening your arms. Keep your head, neck, back, and hips in line as you lift your body off the floor. When your arms are almost fully extended, hold, and then slowly lower yourself back down to the floor.

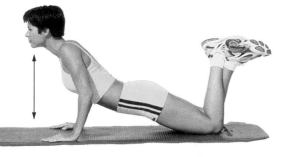

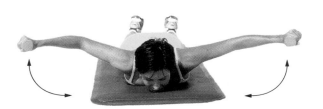

2. Reverse fly: Lie facedown on the floor with a dumbbell in each hand. (You can put a towel under your head for comfort.) Start with your arms out to your sides, palms facing down. Squeezing your shoulder blades together, lift your arms and hands off the floor as high as possible. Hold, and then slowly lower.

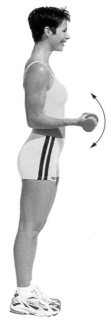

3. Biceps curl:
Stand with your feet shoulder-width apart, holding a dumbbell in each hand. Your arms should be hanging at your sides, palms facing forward. Bending your elbows, raise the dumbbells toward your shoulders. Keep your elbows close to your body. Hold, and then slowly lower.

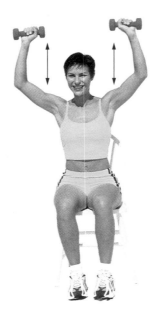

4. Overhead press: Sit tall in a chair with a dumbbell in each hand. Start with your hands at shoulder height, palms facing forward. Raise the dumbbells straight up over your shoulders until your arms are almost fully extended. Hold, and then slowly lower.

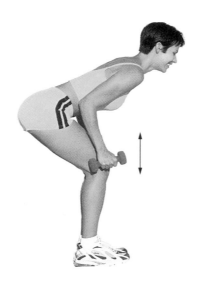

5. Single-arm row: Holding a dumbbell in your right hand, bend forward from your waist and rest your left hand on your knee or a chair. Keep your back flat and knees slightly bent. Your right arm should be hanging straight down, but don't lock that elbow. Bending your elbow, pull the weight straight up toward your chest, keeping your arm close to your body. Hold, and then lower. Repeat on the other side.

For the Lower Body

1. Inner-thigh lift:
Lie on your right side, boosting your upper body on your right elbow and supporting your head on your hand. (If this position bothers your neck, fold your arm down

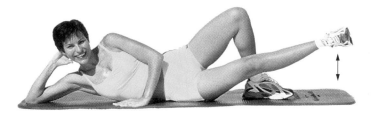

and rest your head on it.) Bend your left leg, placing your foot flat on the floor, keeping your right leg extended and slightly forward. Using your inner-thigh muscles, lift your right leg toward the ceiling at least 6 inches. Hold, and then slowly lower. Repeat on the other side.

2. Outer-thigh
lift: Start in the same position as in the inner-thigh lift, but extend both legs so that they are in line with your body. Slowly lift your top (left) leg to form an 80-degree angle, and then lower. Repeat on the other side.

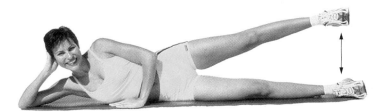

3. Abdominal
crunch: Lie on your back, knees bent, feet flat on the floor and shoulder-width apart. Lightly support your head with your fingertips, elbows out. Press the small of your back into the floor and

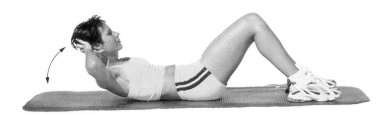

raise your head, shoulders, and upper back off the floor. Keep your abs tight, and keep about a fist-size space between your chin and chest. Come up about 30 degrees, hold, and then slowly lower yourself back down. Don't let your head rest on the floor between reps.

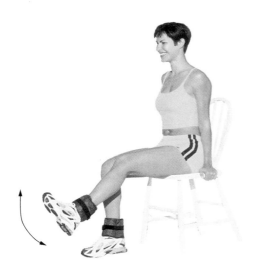 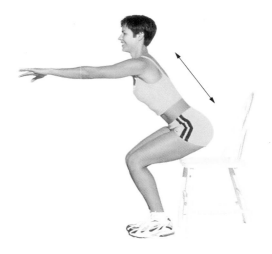

4. Seated leg lift: Wearing ankle weights, sit on a chair or bench with your back straight and feet flat on the floor. Grasp the sides of the chair for balance if needed. Slowly lift your left foot until your calf is in line with your thigh. Hold, and then slowly lower. Repeat with your other leg.

5. Chair squat: Stand with your back to a chair, with your feet a little more than shoulder-width apart. Keeping your hands straight out in front of you for balance, bend at your hips and knees, lowering yourself toward the chair as if you are going to sit. Make sure that your knees do not extend past your toes when you look down, and keep your back straight. Stop before you actually sit. Pause, and then stand back up.

Chapter 13

Drop a Size by Next Month

The *Prevention* 4-Week Fat-Blasting Plan

G ive us 4 weeks, and we'll give you a new body. That's all it takes to see noticeable results: You'll feel stronger and healthier. Have more energy. And best of all, you will be able to slip into a pair of jeans that's one size smaller.

We understand your desire for quick results, so we gathered the best research on healthy ways to lose weight fast and put it into an easy-to-follow plan.

The *Prevention* 4-Week Fat-Blasting Plan will help you burn fat faster, eat 20 percent fewer calories (without feeling hungry), rev up your metabolism, burn more calories in less time, and lose up to 8 pounds! And it's so simple, you can do it anywhere. Get ready, get set, and love your body again.

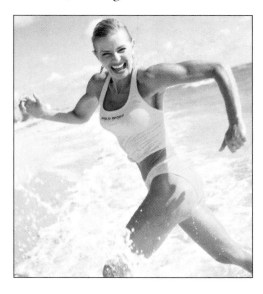

Five-Step Fat-Blasting Diet

Everywhere you look, there's tons of diet advice. We waded through all of that to come up with the five most important steps for dropping pounds fast. Plus, we put together a plan (see "Mix 'n' Match Meals") that makes it easy for you to get started right away.

1. Eat More

Skimpy meals won't satisfy you. "It's the volume of food, not the number of calories you eat, that determines when you're full," says Barbara Rolls, Ph.D., professor at the Pennsylvania State University in University Park and coauthor of *Volumetrics: Feel Full on Fewer Calories*.

"You consistently eat about the same volume of food, day after day. So you can lose weight by eating more low energy density foods: those with

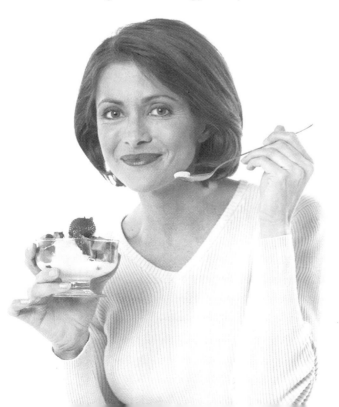

lots of water, such as fruits, vegetables, and broth-based soups," says Dr. Rolls. They help because they're high volume—meaning you get lots of mouthfuls—but low calorie. (High energy density foods, on the other hand, contain loads of calories crammed into a little package.) That's why you can polish off that piece of cheesecake in a snap, but struggle to finish a large salad, notes Dr. Rolls. Eating more low energy density foods can naturally reduce the number of calories you eat by up to 20 percent—without making you feel hungry.

2. Watch Calories

They really do count. But our "Mix 'n' Match Meals" plan does most of the counting for you. You will be able to quickly and easily develop meals to meet your calorie needs. (In general, women should aim for about 1,500 to 1,800 calories a day.)

3. Up the Calcium

Your bones won't be the only things that benefit from this important mineral. People who take in the most calcium (about 1,300 milligrams a day) from food reduce their chances of becoming overweight by an astonishing 80 percent compared to those who eat only 255 milligrams of calcium daily.

According to one recent study with mice, calcium appears to control how fat cells work, say study authors Michael Zemel, Ph.D., and Paula Zemel, Ph.D., of the University of Tennessee-Knoxville. In the study, "mice receiving the most calcium made 51 percent less fat, broke down fat tissue 3 to 5 times faster, and gained up to 40

It's the volume of food, not the number of calories, that determines when you're full.

percent less weight than mice eating the lower calcium diet," he says.

4. Boost Fiber

Upping your fiber intake helps you eat fewer calories, because fiber fills up your tummy faster. Further, fiber blocks absorption of some of the calories you consume by scooting them through your body before they can be absorbed. Experts estimate that each gram of fiber substituted for simple carbohydrates results in a 7-calorie loss. This means that more than tripling your daily fiber intake from 13 grams (the average for most people) to 40 grams (the average for our meal plans) would result in about a 200-calorie deficit a day. This adds up to a 2-pound weight loss in just 1 month.

5. Snack All Day

By eating small meals throughout the day, you'll maximize your body's ability to burn calories. "As you get older, your body's ability to use food decreases," says Julie K. Avery, R.D., a registered dietitian and clinical nutritionist at the Cleveland Clinic Foundation in Ohio. In one study, women whose average age was 72 burned about 30 percent fewer calories after eating a 1,000-calorie meal than younger women whose average age was 25—187 calories versus 246 calories. Both burned similar amounts after 250- and 500-calorie meals. Over time, eating two to three large meals per day (even if you're still eating the same number of calories) could pack on 6 pounds in a year.

Mix 'n' Match Meals

Each day, pick a breakfast, lunch, and dinner from below. Then, depending on your calorie goal, you can have 1 or 2 snacks throughout the day. You should also be drinking about 2 glasses of 2%, 1%, or fat-free milk (86 to 121 calories each, depending on the percentage of fat) a day, and adding a fruit or vegetable to any meal that doesn't already contain one. Also, eat at least one vegetable salad (you can use any of these ingredients: lettuce, peppers, cucumbers, carrots, onions, broccoli, tomatoes, and 2 tablespoons of low-fat dressing) a day.

Breakfast (Average 300 Calories)

Cereal. ½ cup high-fiber cereal with 1 cup fat-free milk and 1 cup fruit

Loaded Omelette. 1 egg + 2 egg whites, ½ cup chopped green bell pepper, and ½ cup chopped mushrooms; 2 slices whole grain toast with 1 teaspoon margarine

Toast. 2 slices of whole grain toast with 2 teaspoons peanut butter and a banana

Egg-Cheese Muffin. 1 poached egg and 1 slice low-fat American cheese on 1 whole wheat English muffin

Whole Wheat Breakfast Cereal. Mix 1 cup cooked bulgur wheat with 2 teaspoons brown sugar, 2 tablespoons chopped dried apricots, and 1 tablespoon chopped walnuts

Raspberry Smoothie. 1 cup low-fat fortified soy milk, 1½ cups frozen raspberries or strawberries (no sugar added), ½ banana, ¼ cup light tofu, and 1 teaspoon sugar (or to taste); mix in blender

Lunch (Average 375 Calories)

Lentil Broccoli Salad. 1 cup chopped romaine lettuce, 1 cup chopped broccoli, ¾ cup cooked lentils (canned is fine; just rinse and drain), and ½ tomato, chopped; Orange-Dill Dressing: mix 1 tablespoon olive oil, 2 tablespoons orange juice, 1 tablespoon fresh chopped dill, ⅛ teaspoon salt, and freshly ground black pepper to taste

Fast Food. Grilled chicken sandwich, extra tomato and extra lettuce, no creamy sauces such as mayo; garden salad with fat-free dressing

Veggie Burger. 1 burger on whole grain hamburger bun with 3 large romaine lettuce leaves, 2 thick tomato slices, and 2 tablespoons honey mustard; small bag of baby carrots

Sandwich. 3 ounces lean turkey breast, ham, or roast beef on 2 slices whole grain bread with 1 ounce 50-percent reduced-fat Cheddar cheese, 1 cup arugula leaves, 2 slices tomato, and 1 tablespoon honey mustard

Pita Egg Salad. Chop 2 cooked egg whites and 1 hard-boiled egg; blend in ¼ cup chopped onion, 2 tablespoons light mayonnaise, 1 tablespoon mustard, and freshly ground black pepper to taste. Cut the top off a 6½-inch whole wheat pita pocket, and stuff with egg mixture, romaine lettuce leaves, and tomato slices.

Easy Tuna Melt. Mix ½ can tuna canned in water with 2 tablespoons light mayo, ¼ cup finely chopped celery, and ¼ cup grated carrot. Divide mixture evenly between two whole wheat English muffin halves. Top each with ½ ounce low-fat Cheddar or low-fat American cheese. Broil until cheese bubbles.

Dinner (Average 475 Calories)

Grilled Maple Marinated Tuna. Marinate a 5-ounce (uncooked portion size) tuna steak in 1½ tablespoons maple syrup, 2 tablespoons orange juice, and freshly ground black pepper for 20 minutes; remove from marinade and grill or broil about 3 minutes on each side.

Medium baked potato topped with 2 tablespoons low-fat sour cream

8 large asparagus spears with 1 teaspoon margarine

Trout Roll-Up. One trout fillet (about 8 ounces, with skin); sprinkle fillet with ¼ teaspoon freshly ground black pepper and ¼ teaspoon salt. Top with ¼ cup chopped green onions. Roll from small end and wrap tightly in aluminum foil. Bake at 350°F for 15 minutes. Remove skin before eating.

1 cup cooked barley

1 cup steamed green beans with 1 teaspoon margarine

Grilled Chicken Dinner.

1 three-ounce grilled chicken breast

1 medium baked sweet potato with 2 teaspoons brown sugar and 1 teaspoon margarine

1 cup spinach with lemon juice

1 whole wheat roll with 1 teaspoon margarine

Ginger-Cilantro Salmon Bake. Spray a 9" × 9" baking dish with vegetable oil spray. Place 3 cups chopped red Swiss chard in bottom. Top with a 5-ounce (raw weight) salmon fillet. Sprinkle with (in the following order) 2 tablespoons chopped fresh ginger, ½ cup chopped green onions, ¼ cup chopped fresh cilantro, and 2 teaspoons soy sauce. Cover tightly with aluminum foil and bake at 350°F for 20 minutes.

Wild Rice–Broccoli Pilaf. Sauté 1 cup chopped broccoli and ½ cup chopped green onion with 1 teaspoon dark sesame oil, 1 clove minced garlic, and dried oregano to taste. When the broccoli is still crisp but tender, blend in ½ cup cooked wild rice.

Mediterranean Pasta. Heat in microwaveable dish about 3 minutes or until heated through: 1 cup frozen broccoli spears, ½ cup white kidney beans, and ½ cup of your favorite jarred pasta sauce. Serve over 1 cup cooked linguine.

Snacks (Average 160 Calories)

Trail Mix. 2 teaspoons dried cranberries; 2 tablespoons raisins; 2 tablespoons peanuts

Veggies and Dip. 10 baby carrots; 1 whole cucumber (sliced); ¼ cup nonfat vegetable dip

Popcorn and Juice. 3 cups light popcorn; 8 ounces calcium-fortified orange juice

Cookies. 3 chocolate chip cookies

Yogurt. 1 cup low-fat yogurt

Fruit Salad. 1 sliced kiwifruit, 1 cup sliced strawberries, and ½ cup blueberries, topped with ¼ cup nonfat whipped topping

¼ Cup Dry-Roasted Peanuts.

1 Ounce Oat Bran Pretzels and ¼ Cup Frozen Yogurt.

Brown Sugar Apple Bagel. ½ whole wheat bagel spread with a mixture of ½ chopped apple blended with 1 tablespoon nonfat cream cheese, 1 teaspoon dark brown sugar, and ¼ teaspoon cinnamon

Three-Step Fat-Blasting Workout

High-intensity workouts are the secret to dropping pounds fast. But don't panic, and don't flip the page thinking, "No way!" A high-intensity workout doesn't necessarily mean you have to run for miles or take an hour-long Spinning class. "Intensity is relative," says Gary Hunter, Ph.D., director of the exercise physiology lab at

"Lose Fat Faster" Workout Schedule

	Interval Workout	Muscle Recovery Workout	Building Workout
Monday	*		
Tuesday		*	*
Wednesday	*		
Thursday		*	*
Friday	*		
Saturday		*	*
Sunday	Rest		

the University of Alabama at Birmingham. "What's high intensity for someone who's unfit may be low intensity for someone who's moderately fit." So no matter what your fitness level, you can get a high-intensity workout by just pushing yourself out of your comfort zone. We'll show you how to do it safely. The results will definitely be worth it.

High-intensity exercise can burn 30 percent to 50 percent more calories than low-intensity exercise. Cycling at a leisurely pace burns about 200 calories in a half-hour, while cycling vigorously burns more than 300.

And the benefits continue even after you stop exercising. After a high-intensity bout of activity, the number of calories you're burning stays elevated for up to 48 hours, which means you could burn an extra 100 calories a day. If you exercise regularly, you could lose an extra pound just from this postworkout calorie burn during the 4-week program.

You'll also become fitter, and moderate-intensity activities will become easier. You'll be able to do more for the same amount of time and effort, meaning you'll burn yet more calo-

HealthPoint

Am I Exercising Too Hard?

Check your heart rate during exercise. An exercise heart rate that is too high (see the guidelines for exercise intensity below) may indicate a problem, says Barry Franklin, Ph.D., president of the American College of Sports Medicine. See your doctor for an exercise stress test if you are at risk for cardiovascular complications such as heart attack, heart disease, angina, respiratory disease, or diabetes; if you have symptoms such as chest pain, pressure, palpitations, or dizziness; or if you have two or more major risk factors for heart disease (smoking, high blood pressure, high cholesterol, obesity, and sedentary lifestyle).

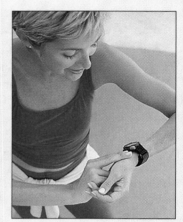

If you have no risk factors, try to get an accurate reading on your heart rate. Take your pulse for 10 seconds instead of 6 for a more accurate count, says Dr. Franklin. For an even more precise measurement, try a heart rate monitor.

Another way to evaluate the intensity of your workout is by perceived exertion. Using a scale of 6 (no effort, such as lounging on the couch) to 20 (very hard, such as sprinting), evaluate how you feel while exercising. You should be around 11 to 13—fairly light to somewhat hard.

Another method is the talk test: While exercising, you should be able to talk well enough to respond to simple questions.

If it still appears that you're working at too high an intensity, ease up. You'll be less likely to suffer muscular or joint injuries—and you will avoid cardiovascular complications if you're at risk.

Age	Heart rate max (beats per min)	Max 10-sec count
35	130–148	22–25
40	126–144	21–24
45	123–140	21–23
50	119–136	20–23
55	116–132	19–22
60	112–128	19–21
65	109–124	18–21

Interval Workout

Start each workout with a 5-minute warmup, then increase to a moderate-intensity bout for the time listed, followed by a high-intensity bout. Repeat those bouts for the number of cycles listed. Finish with a 5-minute cooldown. Total workout time is about 40 minutes.

	Moderate Intensity	High Intensity	Number of Cycles
Week 1	4 min	1 min	6
Week 2	4 min	1½ min	5
Week 3	3 min	2 min	6
Week 4	5 min	5 min	3

ries. For example, if you start out by walking 2 miles in an hour, you'll burn about 160 calories. But as you get fitter, you'll be able to walk 3 miles in an hour for the same effort. You'll burn 50 percent more calories.

Intensity doesn't apply only to aerobic activities. You can burn up to three times as many calories and do fewer repetitions by using a heavier weight when you're strength training.

Here are the three steps to shift your body's calorie-burning engines into overdrive.

Step 1: Interval Workout

By sneaking short, high-intensity bouts of activity into your regular workout, you won't feel like you're killing yourself, and you'll reduce your risk of injury. This 4-week plan will gradually increase the high-intensity portion of your workout, and it can be done with any type of exercise and for any fitness level. During the moderate phase of the workout, you should feel like you're working at an effort of about 6 to 7 (based on a scale from 1 to 10, with 1 being no effort). For the high-intensity phase, you want to push yourself so that you feel like you're at an 8 or 9. At this rate, it should be difficult for you to carry on a conversation. You can do this by going faster, or climbing a hill if you're walking, cycling, or jogging. Swimmers can pick up the pace or do a more difficult stroke. If you're doing step aerobics or kickboxing, increase the intensity with combination arm and leg moves, kicks, jumping jacks, or hops.

Step 2: Recovery workout

This is 30 minutes of aerobic exercise such as walking, jogging, or cycling at a moderate intensity, without the high-intensity intervals. By breaking up your high-intensity workouts with these recovery workouts on alternate days, you'll reduce your risk of injury and prevent burnout. You can choose any activity that you enjoy; just do it at an intensity in which you're breathing a little harder than usual.

Step 3: Muscle-Building Workout

Lifting weights doesn't rate as high as aerobic exercise on the calorie-burn scale. But you can maximize the number of calories you burn while you're lifting by using heavier weights. For this workout (see page 126), aim to use a weight that is heavy enough so that you can do two sets of 8 to 10 reps. The big calorie-burning boost you get from weight training comes after the workout: The muscle you're building burns up to 25 times more calories than fat—all day long.

1. Chest fly: Lying on your back, hold the dumbbells above your chest with your palms facing each other and elbows slightly bent. Lower your arms out to the sides until your upper arms are parallel to the floor. Slowly return to the starting position.

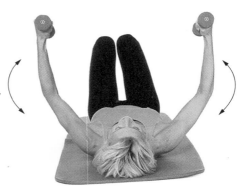

2. Pullover: Lying on your back, hold a dumbbell with both hands above your chest. Lower your arms down and backward over your head as far as possible without discomfort. Don't arch your back. Slowly raise your arms back to the starting position.

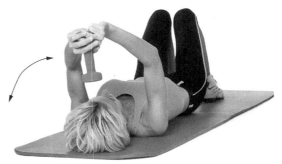

3. Reverse fly: Lie facedown on the floor with a pillow under your chest, a dumbbell in each hand, and your arms out to your sides. Squeezing your shoulder blades, lift your hands off the floor as high as possible. Slowly lower.

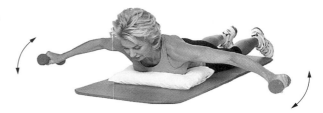

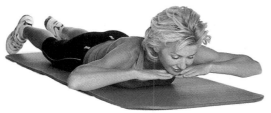

4. Chest lift: Lie facedown on the floor with your hands under your chin. Lift your head and chest off the floor. Slowly lower.

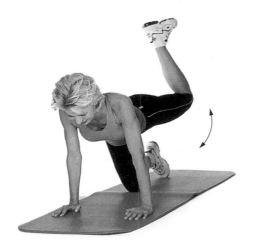

5. Hip extension: Get down on all fours; be sure to keep your back flat. Keeping your knee bent and squeezing your buttocks, lift your left leg up until it is in line with your spine. Slowly lower. Repeat with your right leg.

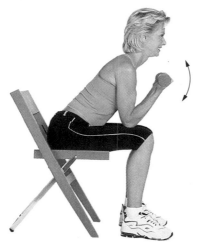

6. Concentrated biceps curl: Sit on a chair and rest your elbows on your knees. Holding a dumbbell in each hand, straighten your arms. Bending your elbows, lift the dumbbells toward your shoulders. Slowly lower.

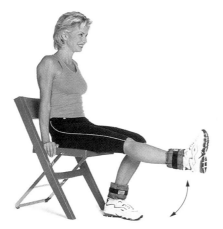

7. Leg extension: Wearing ankle weights, sit on a chair with your feet about hip-width apart. Lift your right foot until it is in line with your thigh. Slowly lower. Repeat with your left leg.

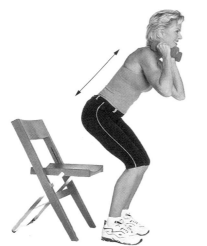

8. Squat: Hold a dumbbell in each hand and curl your arms up to your shoulders. Stand with your back to a chair, with your feet a bit more than shoulder-width apart. Bending at your hips and knees, lower your buttocks toward the chair without touching it. Keep your knees behind your toes. Slowly stand back up.

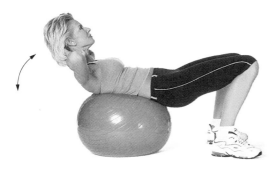

9. Exercise ball crunch: Lie on an exercise ball so that your back is supported and your feet are flat on the floor. With your hands behind your head, curl up, lifting your head, shoulders, and upper back off the ball. Slowly lower.

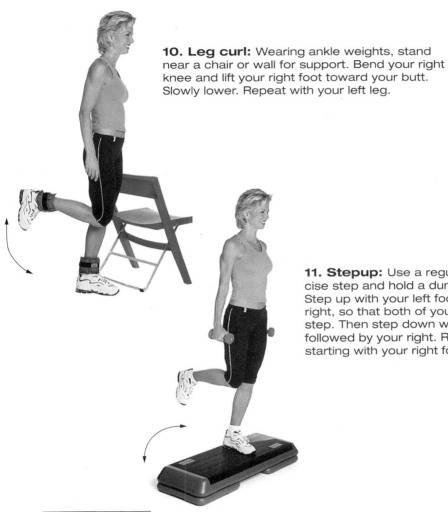

10. Leg curl: Wearing ankle weights, stand near a chair or wall for support. Bend your right knee and lift your right foot toward your butt. Slowly lower. Repeat with your left leg.

11. Stepup: Use a regular step or an exercise step and hold a dumbbell in each hand. Step up with your left foot, followed by your right, so that both of your feet are on the step. Then step down with your left foot, followed by your right. Repeat, this time starting with your right foot.

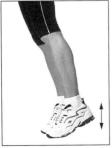

12. Calf raise: Stand with your feet about hip-width apart, holding a dumbbell in each hand. Rise up onto your toes. You may want to hold on to a chair or wall for balance in the beginning. Slowly lower.

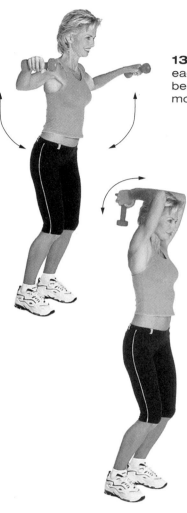

13. Lateral raise: Hold a dumbbell in each hand at your sides. Keeping a slight bend in your elbows, lift the dumbbells almost to shoulder height. Slowly lower.

14. Overhead triceps extension: Hold a dumbbell with both hands over your head. Bending your elbows, lower the dumbbell behind your head. Don't move your upper arms. Slowly raise the dumbell back to the starting position.

LIFESTYLE RESTYLE

Motivated to Move Her Muscles

Nica Russell was certain that she'd never get out of the negative mindset that allowed her weight to escalate to 270 pounds. Then she saw a talk show that completely changed her life.

"Television programs and infomercials about weight loss would bring me to tears, but they couldn't inspire me to get off the sofa and do something," says the 36-year-old Los Angeles resident. "Then I happened to catch an Oprah Winfrey show in which Oprah was crying and talking about her lifelong struggle with her weight. I felt that she was talking directly to me, that she knew exactly how I was feeling. She motivated me to tackle my weight problem."

The next day, Russell went to the nearest mall and headed straight for the video store. She scanned the rows of aerobic-exercise videos and purchased a selection of tapes with workouts ranging from beginner to advanced. Every day for 4 months, in the privacy of her own home, she did a 45-minute video workout. "At first, I could do only about 1 percent of the routines. I felt like I was going to die," she says. "But every time I thought about giving up, I remembered Oprah's words. I found myself going longer without a break and without feeling like passing out. Eventually, I could do my tape routines from beginning to end." At that point, she felt confident enough to visit a gym.

With guidance from a personal trainer at the gym, Russell started lifting weights. Over time, she became an exercise fanatic, working out for 3 hours a day, 7 days a week.

"I was obsessed," she remembers. "But I had a goal to meet." To help her get there, she also made some adjustments in her eating habits, giving up fried foods and filling up on fruits and vegetables. Within 7 months, she lost 135 pounds.

Satisfied with her new, slim physique, Russell began having second thoughts about going to the gym. She was tired of paying the high membership fee, fighting traffic to get there, and waiting in line for equipment. So she decided to create a gym at home.

Over a 2-year period, Russell invested in advanced aerobic-exercise videos, sets of 5- to 25-pound dumbbells, and weight-training equipment with a stairclimber attachment. "My home gym definitely motivates me to stay fit," she says. "Without it, I wouldn't work out as consistently or maintain my weight."

Today, Russell works out for an hour, 4 or 5 days a week. She has maintained her weight at a healthy 135 pounds for 4 years.

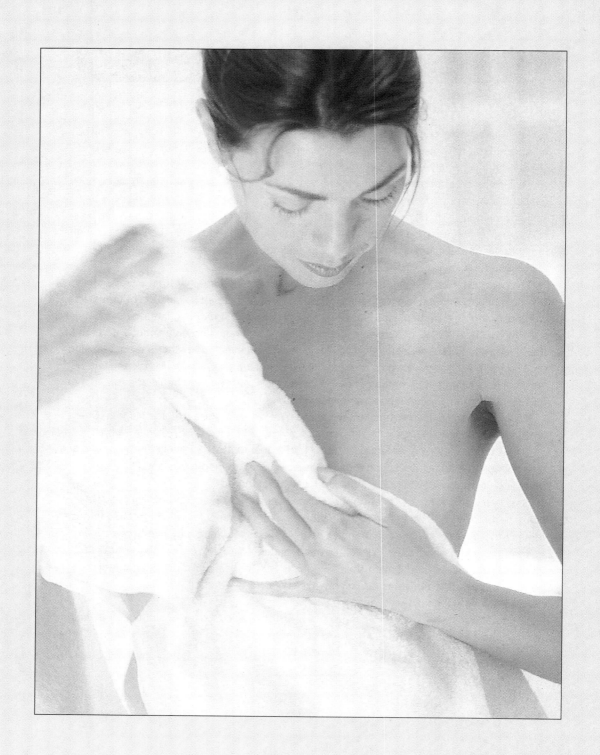

Part Four

Disease Defense
for the
Female Body

Chapter 14

The Year's Top 10 Health Stories

Here's what the latest research means for you.

Most of us get a certain sense of security from the fact that women typically outlive men. According to the National Center for Health Statistics, women can live up to 8 years longer than their male counterparts.

Maybe women live longer because they pay attention to the myriad health tips presented on health-only TV channels, in all those waiting-room magazine articles, and even on the nightly news. Or maybe it's nature; perhaps we simply have a different DNA "destiny."

Regardless of the reasons, we need to be aware of the constantly changing research and how it affects how we approach our daily health regimens. Here are just a few of the leading health issues threatening to steal those precious years away from us.

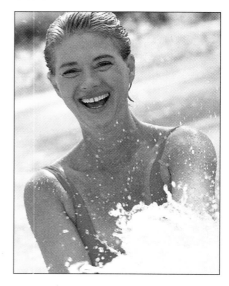

1. Breast Cancer Surgery: Timing Is the Key

According to a British study of 112 women, those who had breast cancer surgery on days 1 or 2 or 13 to 32 of their menstrual cycles had a better survival rate than those who scheduled the procedure on days 3 to 12, when hormones are priming the body for ovulation.

Why? One theory is that during surgery, some cancer cells enter the bloodstream and may be stimulated by the higher estrogen levels that naturally occur before ovulation. If your cycle is regular, it may be possible to schedule surgery during the second half to yield the best benefits and lower the risk of recurrence, says Ruby Senie, Ph.D., a breast cancer epidemiologist and professor of clinical public health in the Mailman School of Public Health at Columbia University in New York City. "But stress can have an impact on the regularity of your menstrual cycle, causing timing to be extremely difficult," she warns. Dr. Senie believes that it's worth discussing with your physician.

2. Estrogen Therapy Minus the Breast Cancer Fears

Researchers have known for some time that use of estrogen-replacement therapy (ERT) for more than 5 to 10 years can increase the average woman's chances of developing breast cancer. As a result, many women steer clear of ERT. But new studies suggest that possibly more of those women may be able to reap ERT's benefits with peace of mind.

Researchers at Vanderbilt University in Nashville studied nearly 10,000 women with a history of noncancerous breast lumps (benign breast disease)—including women with a condition called atypical cell proliferation, which increases breast cancer risk. They found that ERT did not further elevate cancer risk, says lead study author William Dupont, Ph.D., professor of preventive medicine at the university's school of medicine.

A smaller, preliminary study from The University of Texas M. D. Anderson Cancer Center in Houston suggests that ERT may not further increase cancer risk in women with a personal history of breast cancer.

What you can do: If you've been diagnosed with benign breast disease and are interested in ERT, talk to your doctor about these new findings.

If you've been diagnosed with breast cancer, stay tuned—research is ongoing.

3. Get This Lifesaving Test

Because we don't always receive routine cholesterol screenings, women of all ages—as well as men over age 65—are less likely to be treated with drugs to reduce heart attack risk. But a new study suggests that we should.

Researchers at Tulane University Medical Center in New Orleans analyzed five cholesterol-lowering drug studies that included nearly 31,000 people. They found a 30 percent reduction in heart attack risk for both sexes and all age groups receiving the medication.

Because of a lack of research on women and older people, some doctors and insurance companies have been uncertain about whether tests and treatments work for everyone. As a result, some insurers, including Medicare, haven't covered routine cholesterol checks for women and anyone over age 65, says lead researcher John LaRosa, M.D., president of the State University of New York Downstate Medical Center at Brooklyn. This may also explain why fewer women than men are treated with cholesterol-lowering drugs, even though by age 65, women are just as likely to have coronary problems, he says.

Everyone over age 18 should have their cholesterol levels checked at least once every 5 years. Here's what you can do.

Insist on screening and treatment. If the results are high—a total reading higher than 150, with LDL (bad) cholesterol of 130 or higher and HDL (good) cholesterol of 45 or lower—ask your doctor about treatment options, including drugs.

If insurance won't cover it, foot the bill yourself. It's worth it. Cholesterol tests cost an average of $12 to $60. (Watch for advertisements for free screenings, too.) And if your test shows that treatment is necessary, call your insurance company: Test costs may be covered retroactively in this case.

> ## 1-MINUTE FAT BURNER
>
> **Dip your bread. Use olive oil in place of butter. It's healthier and may also help you eat less. In a recent study, dippers ate a total of 52 fewer calories on average than those who used butter.**

This common form of benign uterine tumor is frequently asymptomatic but can cause pelvic pain, anemia, and fertility problems. In the study, those who had the problem reported eating significantly more red meat—and significantly fewer green vegetables—than women who didn't have the tumors.

What's the connection? Excessively high estrogen levels appear to play a role in the development of fibroids—and some research suggests that meat boosts estrogen levels. In addition, a class of compounds called isoflavonoids, found in vegetables and fruits, partly offsets some of estrogen's effects on the body.

About 40 percent of 40-year-old women, and half of 50-year-olds, have clinical (or silent) uterine fibroids.

In light of these findings, you may be able to reduce your odds of developing fibroids (and many other health problems) by following these tips.

• Limit beef, other red meats, and ham. Eat no more than 3 ounces of red meat a day.

• Increase your servings of broccoli, asparagus, spinach, romaine, kale, and other green vegetables. Shoot for at least five servings of vegetables—including one or more servings of the green ones—daily.

4. Prevent Uterine Fibroids with a Color Shift

Italian researchers analyzed the diets of more than 2,300 women, many of whom had fibroids.

5. Eat to Beat Migraine Pain

What's good for the hips and heart may help the head, too. Limiting fat may limit migraine pain, according to a University of California, Irvine, study of 54 migraine-suffering volunteers. After cutting their fat consumption from an average of 66 to 28 grams a day, the participants had fewer, shorter, and less intense migraines. They also needed less migraine medication.

Previous research suggests that certain foods—aged cheeses, nuts, chocolate, red wine and other alcoholic beverages, pea pods, bananas, onions, papaya, and prepared food containing nitrites, monosodium glutamate, or aspartame—can trigger this debilitating headache.

In addition to keeping an eating diary to determine which foods trigger your migraines, you should also limit your fat consumption to roughly 30 grams per day, suggests Merle Diamond, M.D., associate director of the Diamond Headache Clinic in Chicago.

6. Heart Attacks Are Not Just for Men

Women continue to underestimate their risk for heart attack and wait too long to seek medical attention. When researchers recently asked nearly 60 women who had survived heart attacks whether they'd known the warning signs beforehand, more than half said that they hadn't.

Not surprisingly, women who underestimated their heart disease risk had less heart-healthy lifestyles. "We need to more aggressively educate women about heart disease," concludes lead study author Nieca Goldberg, M.D., chief of the women's heart program at Lenox Hill Hospital in New York City and spokesperson for the American Heart Association.

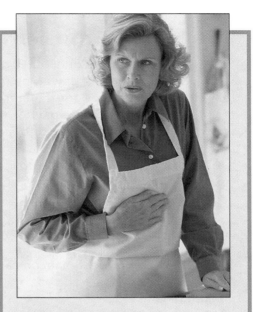

The Ladylike Symptoms of Heart Attack

In men, chest pain and tightness that spreads to the back, neck, shoulders, and arms are typical heart attack warning signs. But one in five women may experience any of the following "atypical" symptoms—and should seek medical attention promptly.

- Severe shortness of breath
- Pain in the upper abdomen (just under the breastbone)
- Nausea or vomiting
- Profound fatigue or weakness
- Unexplained anxiety or a feeling of being unwell
- Profuse sweating

The "Butts Stop Here" Program

1. Start the medication first. Begin 1 to 2 weeks before your quit day. (Most people take a 150-milligram pill for the first 3 to 7 days, then one pill twice a day for 6 to 12 weeks.) Bupropion is believed to stabilize the same brain chemistry that nicotine stimulates, but isn't addictive. It's nicotine-free, so you won't suffer withdrawal symptoms when you stop using it.

*Caution:*Tell your doctor if you have a seizure disorder; this medicine may increase the risk.

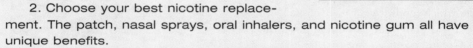

2. Choose your best nicotine replacement. The patch, nasal sprays, oral inhalers, and nicotine gum all have unique benefits.

3. Get professional counseling. Aim for four to seven sessions over a 2-month period, ideally with a clinician specializing in treating addictions.

7. Cream Those Hot Flashes

Does natural progesterone work? Thanks to a new study, there's solid information on what natural progesterone creams applied to the forearm, chest, and upper thigh really can and can't do when massaged into the skin.

Hot flash cooler? YES. After 1 year, more than 80 percent of women using natural progesterone cream reported improvement of their hot flashes, compared with less than 20 percent of those using a placebo, says study author James Anasti, M.D., a reproductive endocrinologist at St. Luke's Hospital in Bethlehem, Pennsylvania. That's good news for the 7 in 10 women who experience hot flashes!

Bone guard? NO. When researchers tested the bone density of 90 postmenopausal women, they discovered no significant differences between those using 20 milligrams per day of the natural progesterone cream and those using a placebo.

Protection against cancer? NO. Doctors generally include synthetic progestins in hormone-replacement therapy (HRT) to protect against a risky buildup of uterine tissue caused by the estrogen. Right now, there's no evidence that progesterone cream offers the same protection against this condition that can lead to uterine cancer. "If you're taking estrogen, I would not recommend this cream in place of oral progesterone," Dr. Anasti says.

8. Quit Smoking for Good

A year after 4,000 fed-up cigarette smokers tried a new, three-part smoke-stopper program, 40 to 60 percent remained smoke-free—a dramatic achievement, compared to the 10 to 15 percent success rate for nicotine-replacement products alone.

With your doctor's help, you can try this effective approach, which combines tailored counseling to explore the reasons why you smoke; the new non-nicotine smoking-cessation pill, bupropion (Zyban); and a nicotine-replacement product, says Linda Hyder Ferry, M.D., chief of preventive medicine at Jerry L. Pettis Veterans Affairs Medical Center in Loma Linda, California.

9. Fight Germs— Without Making Them Stronger

When you feel congested, feverish, and achy, it's tempting to call the doctor and plead for antibiotics. But antibiotics aren't always the solution.

Antibiotics can't help if you have a cold or the flu, since they're caused by viruses. In these cases, the best bet is usually to rest, drink lots of fluids, and, if necessary, take pain relievers for a couple of days.

Moreover, taking antibiotics when you don't need them can contribute to antibiotic-resistant bacteria, which is a growing worldwide health problem. "There are bacteria that live in our sys-tems all the time, and the chance that they will survive antibiotics and develop resistance to them increases every time the bacteria are exposed to the drugs," explains Allan Rosenfield, M.D., dean of the Mailman School of Public Health at Columbia University in New York City.

Of course, antibiotics are essential, even life-saving, when you have a bacterial infection such as strep throat or pneumonia, says Ariel Pablos-Mendez, M.D., assistant professor at Columbia University's schools of medicine and public health in New York City. How do you know whether cold or sore throat symptoms require antibiotics? Follow these general guidelines.

For healthy, young adults:

1. If you have a high fever, whitish spots inside your throat, and swollen glands in your neck, you probably have strep and will need antibiotics. Call your doctor.

2. If you have no signs of strep and no other medical conditions, wait 3 to 4 days. If it's a cold or the flu, you should start feeling better by then. If not, make an appointment to see your doctor.

For the elderly, those with existing breathing problems, or the immune-compromised:

1. Check for strep (see #1 above).

2. If you have chest pain or a lot of phlegm in your respiratory tract, see your doctor immediately.

3. If you have no signs of strep, chest pain, or conges-

Antibotics can't help if you have a cold or the flu, since they're caused by viruses.

tion, call your doctor. Describe your symptoms and ask whether you should go in for a visit.

10. Drop a Little Weight, Feel Great

Annoyed by more aches and pains lately? Feeling pooped? Check the fit of your jeans. Chances are, they've become a little snug. Research suggests that shedding that little bit of extra weight could help ease the aches and restore your zing.

A new Harvard University study of more than 40,000 women has found that gaining as little as 5 to 10 pounds may increase physical pain, while it zaps vitality and physical functioning. Study participants filled out a quality-of-life questionnaire and told researchers about recent weight gain history. Compared to women who lost 5 to 10 pounds, gainers scored lower for physical functioning, vitality, and freedom from bodily pain.

The flip side? Losing even a small amount of weight could help you feel better, both physically and emotionally. "There is compelling evidence that even small to moderate amounts of excess weight affect not only physical health but also your emotional health and quality of life," says JoAnn E. Manson, M.D., professor of medicine at Harvard's Brigham and Women's Hospital in Boston. Here's how to put the loss of a few pounds to work for you.

Strive for and celebrate small losses. Even if you lose only 5 pounds, consider it a victory for your body and your mind.

Keep tabs on weight gain. Disregarding a few extra pounds here and there could add up to serious problems. "Gaining more than 10 to 15 pounds during adulthood is linked to several health risks, including increased risk of hypertension and diabetes as well as a decline in the quality of life," Dr. Manson says.

Make small, easy changes for big results. To lose a moderate amount of weight, or to keep a small weight gain from growing into a bigger one, concentrate on simple lifestyle changes. "As little as 30 minutes of brisk walking a day and cutting back on calories can do it. It doesn't require a starvation diet," Dr. Manson says. Increase the amount of fruits, vegetables, and whole grains in your diet, and you'll naturally cut back on calories.

Chapter 15

Your Healthy-Heart Program

It takes more than diet and exercise to prevent a heart attack.

No matter who's doling it out, heart-healthy advice usually goes something like this: Stop smoking; cut down on fat; and exercise, exercise, exercise. It's the rare doctor who also tells you: Have some fun. Put a little love in your heart. Focus on friendships. Practice positive thinking.

Well, consider yourself told. Because new medical research suggests that your mental attitude plays a major role in helping you recover from a heart attack and avoid that first one. It turns out that negative emotions like anger, loneliness, and stress can harm your heart. To prevent them from doing any damage, you need to gain control over them.

You literally need "a change of heart."

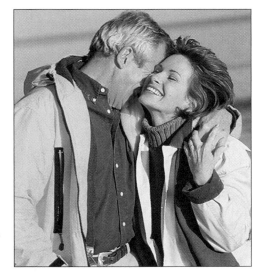

Feeling Bad Puts You at Risk

A recent study found that being even mildly depressed after a heart attack can double your risk of dying from another. Even if you haven't had a heart attack, stress and distress increase your risk of having one, too. A long-term study of more than 900 Finnish men ages 42 to 60 found that, over the course of about 4 years, the carotid artery walls of those who characteristically reacted most strongly to stress were thicker than those who handled stress well. Thickened blood-vessel walls pose an increased risk for heart attack.

How do you lighten up? Mood-altering medications such as fluoxetine (Prozac) can help. But research also shows that modifying your behavior—your response to depression and other negative emotions—can also go a long way to attack-proofing your heart. Here are the best ways to regain control.

Try Psychotherapy

Forget that picture you have of a pointy-bearded mind-mender taking you all the way back to the trauma of toilet training. Not all psychotherapy is that probing. Many therapists take a much more immediate, practical approach.

"The form of psychotherapy that most people agree is best to use is cognitive behavior therapy," says Redford B. Williams, M.D., chief of behavioral medicine at Duke University in Durham, North Carolina, and coauthor of *Lifeskills*. Cognitive therapy helps you learn to make more rational and accurate assessments of your thoughts and feelings in life's tough situations. That's important because if you're depressed, you're likely to interpret everything as being hopeless and will see other people's actions as confirmation that there must be something wrong with you.

Make Friends

Loneliness can shorten your life. A recent study of 292 people hospitalized for clinical heart failure found that those who were socially isolated were much more likely than their more socially well-connected peers to experience a fatal cardiac event or to be readmitted for a heart problem such as angina or heart failure. Although the study examined both men and women, the effect was most pronounced in women.

Lead author Harlan M. Krumholz, M.D., associate professor of medicine at Yale University School of Medicine, believes that the women may have suffered because isolation made their hearts more prone to the hormonal effects of stress, and the women were less likely to care for themselves when they felt that no one else cared for them.

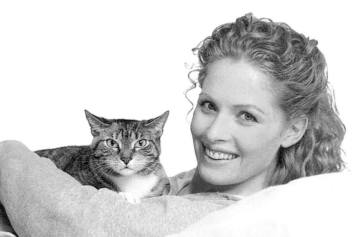

Studies show that owning **a pet can help you follow through** with cardiac rehabilitation.

Eight Ways to Prevent a Heart Attack

1. Don't smoke.
2. Eat a diet that gets 25 percent of its calories from fat, 60 to 65 percent from carbohydrates, and 10 to 15 percent from protein, with 25 to 35 grams of fiber.
3. Walk the equivalent of 2 miles a day most days.
4. Lose weight if you're overweight. One reliable indicator of where you stand is the body mass index (BMI). To calculate your BMI, use the information found in "Lose Weight, Not Your Gallbladder" on page 3.
5. Decrease your saturated fat intake to no more than 20 grams daily (10 grams if you've had a heart attack).
6. Decrease your dietary cholesterol to no more than 300 milligrams daily (200 milligrams if you've had a heart attack).
7. If you're postmenopausal, discuss hormone-replacement therapy (HRT) with your physician.
8. Regularly practice stress-reduction techniques.

Regardless of the underlying mechanism, what's most revealing about this study is that loneliness, like anger, kills. "In this population of heart patients, this social isolation rivaled any other type of predictor, including impaired heart function," says Dr. Krumholz. "There were no other factors that were substantially more important."

If you don't have family and friends living near you, you can join a support group. Depressed Anonymous is an international 12-step organization that can help you deal with the blues. For information about this organization, send a SASE to Depressed Anonymous, P.O. Box 17471, Louisville, KY 40217 or visit their Web site at www.depressedanon.com.

If you've had a heart attack, try Mended Hearts, a national organization offering information and support to people with heart disease. Call them at the American Heart Association (800-242-8721) or check their Web site at www.mendedhearts.org.

Get a Pet

Studies show that people who own pets have significantly lower blood pressure than people who don't own pets. There's even evidence that people at high risk of heart attack because they're hostile have fewer dangerous physical reactions to stress when they have a dog by their side for comfort.

But Rover or Puff can mean even more to

your health if you've had a heart attack. A University of Texas at El Paso study showed that pet owners were far more likely to complete a course of cardiac rehabilitation (96 percent) than those who had no furry friends (77 percent).

Why? A dog or cat might be just the reason you need to get out of bed—and get better. Owning a pet, Dr. Williams suggests, provides "a source of nonjudgmental, unalloyed social support." That's doctor talk for unconditional love.

Meditate

Meditation isn't just for Benedictine monks. In fact, the mindfulness and sense of peace engendered by meditation have heart-healthy benefits for everyone, according to John Astin, Ph.D., a postdoctoral fellow and stress management consultant at the Preventive Cardiology Clinic at Stanford University School of Medicine.

Exactly how meditation relieves stress isn't entirely clear. In some cases, it may work directly through its calming effects on the cardiovascular and hormonal systems. As research by Herbert Benson, M.D., head of the Mind/Body Medical Institute at Harvard Medical School and Beth Israel Hospital in Boston, suggests, techniques such as meditation may produce what he refers to as the relaxation response, which counteracts or balances the fight-or-flight response that puts strain on the heart when repeatedly activated.

Meditation, particularly certain forms such as mindfulness meditation, can also teach you new ways to respond to the negative effects of stress in a calmer way, suggests Dr. Astin. You learn to simply observe powerful thoughts and emotions that arise in response to stress without having to automatically react.

For example, instead of having a knee-jerk, full-blown, hormone-pumping response to a stressor—yelling and honking at the guy who

Bad Feelings Can Break Your Heart

Though little is known about the effects of emotions on your heart, there are a few theories about why negative feelings can do so much damage.

It could be physical: Stress and depression can ratchet up the levels of certain hormones, says Redford B. Williams, M.D., chief of behavioral medicine at Duke University in Durham, North Carolina, and coauthor of *Lifeskills*. One of those hormones, adrenaline, can trigger abnormal heart rhythms. Another, norepinephrine, is blamed for a multitude of sins, such as raising blood pressure and cholesterol. A third hormone, cortisol, can do all of the above and shut down your immune system.

Or it could be psychological: Heart attack survivors who are anxious, angry, or depressed may be less motivated to do the things they need to do to become long-term survivors. They may be less likely to eat a more heart-healthy diet, get regular exercise, or take medication.

just cut you off on the highway—you can "step back" and decide that it's better to have a bad driver in front of you so you can keep an eye on him. In any case, it's your decision.

Check your local hospital or adult night school for meditation or tai chi courses. (There's a meditative aspect to tai chi, a gentle form of the Chinese martial arts.) Other resources include tapes and books, such as *The Relaxation Response* by Dr. Benson, which teaches one of the simplest and most medically proven forms of meditation.

Put a Little Love in Your Heart

Rollin McCraty, director of research for the Institute of HeartMath in Boulder Creek, California, and his staff teach people how to use love and appreciation to heal their hearts.

That approach is the centerpiece of the institute's pioneering techniques, one of which is called Freeze Frame. This technique prompts you to recognize the signs of stress and "freeze"—take a timeout—instead of reacting to it. The best news? You don't have to travel to California to try it.

When you find yourself in a stressful situation, shift your focus to the area around your heart and hold your attention there for at least 10 seconds as though you were breathing through your heart. Then, recall a positive feeling and re-experience it.

"In the beginning, you can do it by recalling a time in your life when you were feeling really good, really appreciating something," explains McCraty. When stress hits, think of something that stirred those appreciative emotions—anything from the birth of your first child to hearing the Boston Pops play the 1812 Overture.

That powerful positive emotion shifts the

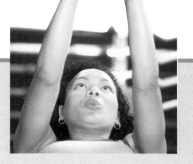

Beat Stress the Easy Way

A heart-pounding workout may seem like a good way to vent frustration, but it may not be the best choice if you're not typically active. When 12 sedentary people exercised at various intensities, researchers found that anxiety decreased during the lowest-intensity exercise (equivalent to an easy walk).

Anxiety levels also dropped when individuals were able to choose their preferred workout level. "They may have had more self-confidence when they controlled the intensity," says study author Jeffrey Pasley, of the University of Georgia in Athens.

If you're not active, here's how to get the most stress relief from activity.

- Keep the pace easy and comfortable.
- Don't take a class or exercise with someone who will push you too hard.
- Do something you enjoy.

rhythmic pattern of the heart and can favorably alter a number of bodily functions, including your blood pressure.

The next step, he says, is to "ask your heart or your intuition—whatever you call it— what would be a more efficient response to the situation." You may be surprised at what you come up with in that more positive state of mind. It's hard to respond with anger, for example, when the thought of your newborn makes you smile. "Then," says McCraty, "listen to what your heart says and follow up on what that tells you."

Sound a little far out? Cardiologists don't

Weight Loss
HELP OR HYPE?

Log On, Lose Weight

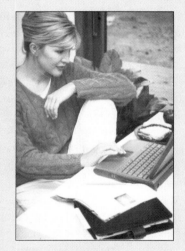

Sitting at a computer may help you slim down. Research has already shown that support groups help you keep pounds off. Now, a new study indicates that online support groups work, too.

After a 15-week weight-loss program, dieters who got online support to help maintain their slimmer figures actually lost an additional 3½ pounds on average. (A group who attended bi-weekly meetings lost about the same amount.)

"You need to find other dieters who share common experiences," explains study author Jean Harvey-Berino, Ph.D., of the University of Vermont in Burlington. "The Internet allows you to do that easily." It's a great tool if you don't have time to attend meetings, don't have any weight-loss groups nearby, don't like talking in groups, or need help when late-night munchies hit.

Here are two exceptional Web sites to help you.

• www.prevention.com. For great tips and practical advice for dieters, visit *Prevention*'s site on the Web.

• www.3fatchicks.com. Four years ago, three overweight sisters started this site to chronicle their weight-loss obstacles and successes. What has evolved is a fun site full of resources that can inspire your weight-loss efforts.

think so. McCraty's research has been published in major cardiology journals, and doctors refer patients to the institute for help in learning to deal with their turbulent emotions. Most have a successful change of heart. Says McCraty: "We've had people here who were literally able to stop arrhythmias." For more information, visit their Web site at www.heartmath.com.

Say Your Prayers

Whether or not faith moves mountains, belief in a higher power can move you, according to Dr. Williams. "Leave out the secular benefits (socialization), and there may be something there from God. Who knows? But it's well-known that people who are more actively religious are healthier."

When you think about it, this isn't so far-fetched. Just like meditating and calming erratic emotions, "having" religion or relying on a higher power as a support can be very positive. People who believe in God expect great things, and so having faith is often equated with having a great sense of hope. Hope gives you something to hold on to and to get you through stressful and turbulent situations.

Get In Touch with Your Natural Rhythms

Biofeedback might sound a little bit "out there," sort of like mood rings, but the science behind the technology is well-established. You can use it to learn a stress-reduction technique that can help you lower your cardiovascular risk factors.

In one study conducted by researchers at the University of California, Los Angeles, chronic heart failure patients were able to improve their bloodflow in 20-minute biofeedback sessions. The 40 study participants were shown readings

of their skin temperatures and asked to raise them by thinking about calm, soothing settings and imagining warmer hands. Not only did they increase bloodflow, their breathing rates were also lower.

To find a certified biofeedback practitioner near you, send a SASE to the Biofeedback Certification Institute of America, 10200 West 44th Avenue, Suite 304, Wheat Ridge, CO 80033 or visit the organization's Web site at www.bcia.org.

It's important to note that biofeedback, and the rest of these techniques, should not be considered a substitute for standard medical treatment, but rather an additional tool.

The Fastest Way to Your Heart Is through Your Mind

Which approach or technique is best for you? It's really a personal choice. Of course, no approach is helpful if you don't recognize that you have a problem and that you need help. For that reason, Dr. Williams recommends thorough mental health evaluations for patients following a heart attack.

The emotional component of heart disease, Dr. Williams contends, "has been unappreciated." Depression, in particular, is often overlooked. Even if it is recognized, it usually goes untreated.

"But the failure to recognize and deal with such devastating psychic pain could have disastrous results," warns Dr. Williams. After all, he says, depression "won't just make you miserable, it can kill you." But you don't have to let it if you follow our mind-healing strategies for a healthier heart.

Chapter 16

One Vitamin Cures Your Cholesterol Problems

Niacin: It's the miracle heart remedy that doctors ignore.

If your cholesterol level is starting to look like a pretty good bowling score, your doctor has probably given you two choices: One, clean up your act and your arteries by eating right and exercising. And two, if you need more help, take cholesterol-lowering drugs—very likely one of the widely prescribed "statins" such as simvastatin (Zocor) or atorvastatin (Lipitor).

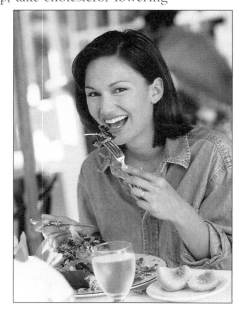

What your doctor may not tell you is that you have a third, all-but-forgotten option: to take the B vitamin known as niacin. In fact, experts at some of the nation's top heart centers are now saying that niacin could be your very best choice, depending on your individual cholesterol profile. That's why this amazing remedy seems primed for a comeback.

What You Need to Know about Cholesterol

Until recently, the big focus in cholesterol control was reducing your low-density lipoproteins (LDL), a form of cholesterol known to clog your arteries. Statins lower LDL more than any other cholesterol-lowering drug—by 20 to 60 percent—which explains their popularity. No wonder doctors have been prescribing them like gangbusters: From January to November 1999, statins accounted for 89 percent of all cholesterol-lowering prescriptions.

That's great if high LDL is your only problem. But today, we know there are two more major "lipid subfractions," as they are called, that can also raise your risk of a heart attack if they're out of line.

High-density lipoproteins (HDL). This is a "good" cholesterol that, like a detergent, scours "bad" LDL cholesterol away from artery walls.

Triglycerides. These are the noncholesterol fats in your blood, which are also linked to heart disease at high levels.

What if, like many others, you find that your HDL and triglyceride levels aren't what they should be? Experts agree that you can't ignore them. "Controlling all of the lipid subfractions is vital when it comes to fighting heart disease," says cholesterol researcher Antonio Gotto, M.D., dean of the Weill Medical College at Cornell University in New York City.

Take HDL, the good cholesterol. According to a recent study, only about 20 percent of people who have heart attacks have high LDL only. Researchers estimate that 25 percent of those who develop heart disease have low HDL. "There is a substantial amount of epidemiological evidence that suggests that HDL is just as important as LDL when it comes to predicting your cardiac risk," says researcher Greg Brown, M.D., Ph.D., professor of cardiology at the University of Washington in Seattle.

Do You Have the Wrong Number?

The American Heart Association (AHA) considers a total blood cholesterol level between 200 and 239 to be borderline-high, and above 240 to be high. Many doctors have tougher goals for their patients; for instance, they may view anything above 200 as high. Period. *Prevention*'s goal is even tougher: below 150.

Here are the AHA recommendations for lipid subfractions—and *Prevention*'s tougher guidelines.

LDL: Below 160 if you have no more than one risk factor (such as smoking or diabetes) or less than 130 if you have two or more risk factors. *Prevention*'s goal: below 130 for everyone.

HDL: Greater than 35. *Prevention*'s goal: greater than 45.

Triglycerides: Less than 200. *Prevention*'s goal: 150—or less than 100 if you've had a heart attack.

How a B Vitamin Can Help You

This is where niacin comes in. "It's the only drug on the market that improves all the measures of cholesterol," says William B. Parsons Jr., M.D., author of *Cholesterol Control without Diet! The Niacin Solution* and one of the doctors who first discovered the cholesterol-lowering potential of niacin in the 1950s.

While statins work primarily on LDL, studies show that niacin works on everything: LDL drops by 10 to 25 percent, triglycerides plummet 20 to 50 percent, and HDL soars upward 15 to 35 percent. In daily doses of 1,000 to 3,000 milligrams (50 to 150 times higher than the Daily Value for niacin and far higher than you could get from food), it becomes a drug that can improve your whole lipid profile—dramatically.

True, the effect of the statins on LDL is greater, and they modestly raise HDL. "But niacin regulates all of the lipid subfractions, especially HDL, in the right direction," says David Capuzzi, M.D., Ph.D., director of the Cardiovascular Disease Prevention Center at Thomas Jefferson University Hospital in Philadelphia. "Niacin does all the right things."

Another niacin advantage: It's cheap. "Many patients can't afford to take their cholesterol medications because currently, they're expensive," says Dr. Capuzzi. Statins cost $2 to $3.50 for one tablet. But Niaspan, one of the most expensive forms of niacin, costs just under $1 per tablet.

The Other Side of Niacin

Right about now, you're probably asking yourself, "If niacin is so great and cheap to boot,

Change Your Diet

You can actually lower your total cholesterol by as much as 40 percent through diet alone. Here's how.

- Eat a diet that gets no more than 25 percent of daily calories from fat; 60 to 65 percent from carbohydrates; and 10 to 15 percent from protein.
- Aim for five servings of vegetables and four servings of fruit daily.
- Choose low-fat or fat-free dairy products.
- Limit your intake of low-fat meats and poultry to 3 ounces or less a day.
- Increase your fiber intake to 25 to 35 grams a day.
- Eat fewer refined foods and more whole grains.

why aren't more doctors recommending it?"

It's partly because niacin has an undeserved bad reputation. Many doctors turned away after a highly publicized 1994 study concluded that serious liver side effects were too common with niacin. Unfortunately, that study used higher-than-recommended doses. More recent research has established that liver complications from niacin given at proper doses occur infrequently—in less than 1 percent of patients in Dr. Brown's research. With the statins, liver side effects occur at about the same rate, according to the National Heart, Lung, and Blood Institute (NHLBI).

As a result, whether you're taking a statin or niacin, your doctor should monitor your liver enzymes—every 6 weeks to 3 months for the first year, less often after that—so that the dose can be modified or discontinued at the first sign of any trouble, before damage is done.

Because other side effects from niacin may include high blood sugar and gout, your doctor may not prescribe niacin if you have diabetes or high uric acid levels.

It Turns On the Heat

The other big reason that doctors snub niacin is because getting the patient started requires a little coaching. Initially, most people who take niacin experience flushing, which, like a hot flash, feels and looks like mild sunburn and usually occurs in the face, and sometimes in the chest. Depending on which form of niacin you take, it can start 10 to 30 minutes after you take it and last about 10 minutes.

"I think that in many cases, a physician will prescribe niacin, the patient will take one pill, experience flushing, and will want to quit," says Dr. Brown.

But here's the big advantage to riding out niacin's side effects: The symptoms will usually subside as your body adjusts to niacin therapy. According to Dr. Brown's research, within a few weeks, 80 to 90 percent of patients tolerate niacin well when it's taken in moderate amounts. The research also indicates that flushing can be eliminated 80 percent of the time by taking niacin with meals; by avoiding alcohol, spicy foods, and hot liquids; and by not skipping doses.

Minimize Your Problems

Starting on a low-dose form of niacin and gradually increasing the dosage over 6 to 8 weeks will help diminish flushing. So can experimenting with different forms.

Another option: The prescription niacin called Niaspan is designed to be taken before bed, so that when flushing occurs, you're asleep. If flushing is bothersome, taking an aspirin with or before your niacin may help until your body adjusts and flushing episodes settle down. Aspirin suppresses the activity of blood vessel chemicals called prostaglandins, which produce the flushing.

The bottom line: Your doctor might be omitting a key option in cholesterol control because he's overlooking the two critical components when it comes to niacin therapy: persistence and patience.

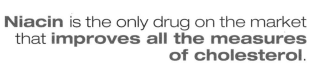

Niacin is the only drug on the market that **improves all the measures of cholesterol**.

Are You a Perfect Candidate?

Whether or not niacin, a statin, or even both are right for you depends on your cholesterol profile. "If all you have is a high LDL problem that isn't responding to lifestyle changes, then a statin probably is the answer for you," says Dr. Gotto. "But if you need a correction to the other subfractions, you should talk to your doctor about other cholesterol-lowering options."

What if all your levels are in the danger zone: Your LDL is high, your HDL is low, and your triglycerides are high? Then you may be a perfect candidate for niacin. The NHLBI describes niacin as "the drug of first choice" for patients in this category.

If your levels are extremely high, you and your doctor might also want to consider what's referred to as combination therapy, a strategy some experts consider the wave of the future. Combination therapy is a statin plus niacin, or a statin plus niacin plus another lipid-lowering drug, such as a fibrate.

"A lot of the leading lipid clinics are now using combination therapy because they know it works," says Dr. Brown. By combining statin and niacin therapies, he says, patients enjoy as much as double the usual 30-percent reduction in heart attack risk that they'd get from one cholesterol-lowering drug alone.

Research does suggest that combination therapy increases your chances of developing

1-MINUTE FAT BURNER

Sprinkle flax on your cereal. High-fiber, ground flaxseed can help curb your appetite and eliminate calories. In addition, the fiber can help lower your total cholesterol level.

liver complications or myopathy, a breakdown of muscle proteins in your body. (A red flag would be flulike symptoms.)

But, says Dr. Brown, if a patient is aware that nausea, vomiting, and muscle aches may be a sign of niacin toxicity, and she is being monitored by a skilled physician, the odds of these problems developing undetected are slim.

One note: Though heart experts experienced in combination therapy are enthusiastic, and though combination therapy is endorsed by the NHLBI and the American Heart Association, its use has not been approved by the FDA, which believes that more study is needed.

How to Take It

You can buy niacin over-the-counter, but you should never decide to take it on your own. Always and only take niacin under a doctor's supervision. At the doses of niacin needed to regulate cholesterol (about 1,000 to 3,000 milligrams), there is a small but real possibility of moderate or severe liver toxicity. Your doctor will run periodic blood tests and check you to determine if you need to stop or reduce the dose for safety reasons, just as he would monitor you if you were taking a statin. There are also prescription versions of niacin, which doctors increasingly prefer. Many doctors are prescribing the newest FDA-approved niacin, Niaspan, which can be taken in one bedtime

Shopping for Niacin

So you've decided to give niacin a try—under your doctor's supervision, of course. Niacin is not a do-it-yourself drug.

What kind do you reach for? If you buy over-the-counter (OTC) niacin to lower your cholesterol, make sure you get the variety called nicotinic acid. There's another type of niacin on store shelves, called nicotinamide or niacinamide, that has no effect on cholesterol.

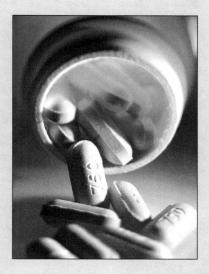

It's best to go with the dosage level your doctor recommends as well as the specific brand or form, since quality can vary. Here are your basic options.

Immediate-release. It's absorbed by your body in minutes. Depending on the brand, it's available OTC or by prescription. It's more likely to cause flushing, but less likely to cause liver complications. The cost is $10 to $20 a month. Dosage: usually three times a day, with bland food.

Extended-, sustained-, slow-, or timed-release. These forms of niacin take several hours to be absorbed by your body. They're available OTC or by prescription. (Two well-known OTC brands are Endur-acin and Slo-Niacin.) They are less likely to cause flushing, but may be more likely to cause stomach upset and liver complications. The cost is about $10 a month. Dosage: depending on the preparation used, usually once or twice a day.

Niaspan. Also considered extended-release, this prescription form of niacin is one of the most popular with doctors. Advantages: You take it only once a day at bedtime, and studies show that it reduces your odds of side effects—from flushing to liver complications. It costs about $30 a month (still a bargain compared to statins). Dosage: nightly, with a bedtime snack.

No-flush. Also called inositol hexanicotinate, it's sold in health food stores and is popular in Europe. Some doctors say they've had great success because it lowers cholesterol without causing flushing; other docs say it hasn't been tested in well-controlled human trials. The jury is still out. It costs about $20 a month. Dosage: several times a day.

A Cholesterol Test at Home?

Should you purchase one of the home tests that is available for keeping tabs on your cholesterol levels? Some experts say not to bother. These tests don't provide your doctor with information that can have a direct impact on your care.

"My big concern is that these tests give you only total cholesterol," says *Prevention* advisor and cardiologist Bernadine Healy, M.D. "They don't tell you your high-density lipoproteins (HDL)." Without your HDL information, there's no way for you or your doctor to calculate your total cholesterol/HDL ratio, the number that's most important when evaluating your risk. This is especially problematic for many women, who, at first glance, have total cholesterol levels that are too high. Only by checking the total cholesterol/HDL ratio can a woman know if she's truly at increased risk for heart disease.

dose, is well-tolerated, and has been proven safe and effective.

Your best bet: Find a doctor who is "good at niacin," says Dr. Parsons. That means someone who can discuss with you what niacin has to offer. If the two of you decide that niacin is right for you, take the version that your doctor recommends, and follow all directions carefully.

Chapter 17

How Strong Are Your Bones, Really?

You and your doctor may be missing the boat on bone health.

A national survey of 1,000 women ages 30 and older conducted by *Prevention* magazine found that women and their doctors are sorely misinformed about osteoporosis. Even worse, many women aren't taking even the most basic steps to reduce their risks.

Seven out of 10 women say that their doctors have never talked to them about osteoporosis, though half of them women will break a bone because of osteoporosis sometime after age 50. More than half of those women say that their doctors have never recommended a bone-density test.

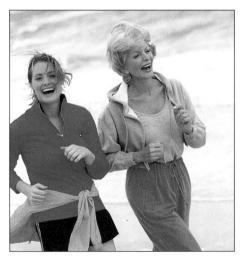

Only 11 percent of the women surveyed think that it's very likely that they will get osteoporosis, even though one in five women can expect to develop the disease.

Ignorance Isn't Bliss

Ignorance about osteoporosis is dangerous. Not only is this bone-thinning disease deadly (complications from hip fracture kill about 35,000 people a year), it's a major crippler of women. It can rob you of your independence: your ability to walk, play with your grandchildren, cook for yourself, plant flowers in the spring, even climb into the tub for a relaxing bubble bath.

The most serious complication of osteoporosis is hip fracture. Only one-third of all people who fracture their hips ever fully recover. It often means a prolonged stay in a nursing home. But for as many as one in five, it may mean death within 1 year.

Half of the women surveyed believe that a severe case of osteoporosis would interfere with their daily activities. But in reality, even a moderate case, characterized by stooped posture, chronic back pain, and height loss, can make everyday movements, such as hooking your bra or enjoying a walk, a luxury of the past.

Nothing Fits!

It doesn't take a hip fracture to change the quality of your life. "Many women fear changes in their appearance as they age," says John Bilezikian, M.D., director of the metabolic bone diseases program at Columbia–Presbyterian Medical Center in New York City. "But if they were aware of the changes to their appearance with osteoporosis, they might take this disease more seriously."

The loss of height that you experience with osteoporosis is caused when the vertebrae in your spine become so thin that they begin to collapse under the weight of your own body. There isn't enough room for your internal organs, so they push out, creating a bulging stomach. "Your clothes won't fit anymore," says Dr. Bilezikian. "They'll hang unevenly if you develop curvature of the spine due to the collapsing vertebrae."

Test Your Bone Smarts

Do you think you know enough about your bone health? Here's a way to find out. Place a check next to every bone fact that you know, then compare your knowledge to that of women who participated in a *Prevention* magazine osteoporosis survey.

☐ **A broken bone after age 50 is a symptom of osteoporosis.** *Forty-seven percent of the women over 50 didn't know that a broken bone is a symptom of osteoporosis.*

☐ **If your mother and/or grandmother had osteoporosis, you're likely to get it.** *Only 38 percent of the women knew that family history was a risk factor for the disease. Worse yet, only 24 percent of the women whose mothers or grandmothers had osteoporosis thought that they were at high risk—and only a little over half*

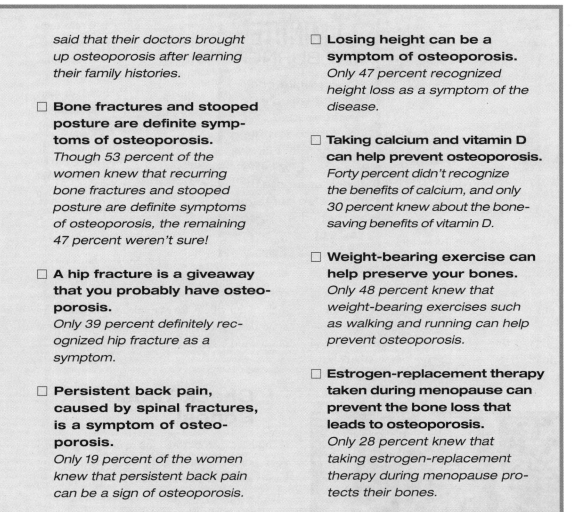

said that their doctors brought up osteoporosis after learning their family histories.

☐ **Bone fractures and stooped posture are definite symptoms of osteoporosis.**
Though 53 percent of the women knew that recurring bone fractures and stooped posture are definite symptoms of osteoporosis, the remaining 47 percent weren't sure!

☐ **A hip fracture is a giveaway that you probably have osteoporosis.**
Only 39 percent definitely recognized hip fracture as a symptom.

☐ **Persistent back pain, caused by spinal fractures, is a symptom of osteoporosis.**
Only 19 percent of the women knew that persistent back pain can be a sign of osteoporosis.

☐ **Losing height can be a symptom of osteoporosis.**
Only 47 percent recognized height loss as a symptom of the disease.

☐ **Taking calcium and vitamin D can help prevent osteoporosis.**
Forty percent didn't recognize the benefits of calcium, and only 30 percent knew about the bone-saving benefits of vitamin D.

☐ **Weight-bearing exercise can help preserve your bones.**
Only 48 percent knew that weight-bearing exercises such as walking and running can help prevent osteoporosis.

☐ **Estrogen-replacement therapy taken during menopause can prevent the bone loss that leads to osteoporosis.**
Only 28 percent knew that taking estrogen-replacement therapy during menopause protects their bones.

‖ Why Didn't I Know This?

Considering that it's such a devastating disease, why are women so misinformed about osteoporosis? Many experts believe that it's because their doctors are misinformed, too. Until recently, there was little doctors could do. Diagnostic tools have been widely available only in the past 5 years, which means that most treatments are relatively new.

"Doctors are only beginning to learn how to deal with osteoporosis in the same way that they now deal with heart disease," explains Robert Lindsay, M.D., Ph.D., immediate past president of the National Osteoporosis Foundation (NOF).

"You don't see bone loss. Since it doesn't cause any problems until a fracture occurs, in many ways, it's similar to where we were with heart disease 10 years ago, when we didn't recognize people with it until they had a heart attack. Now we understand the role of cholesterol in creating plaque buildup in coronary arteries."

Dr. Lindsay estimates that "the average primary care physician sees about 10 or 11 patients every week who have osteoporosis. But doctors are so busy dealing with the problem that the patient came to see them for, that they don't look for or recognize the unseen bone loss."

Also, those physicians who went to medical school 10 or more years ago simply didn't learn much about osteoporosis. Thus, it's off their radar.

While it might be understandable that pri-

> ## 1-MINUTE FAT BURNER
>
> **Pour a white cocktail of fat-free milk because it adds calcium to fortify your bones. Like water, the volume fills your stomach, but it also contains carbohydrates, so you eat less.**

mary care physicians miss signs of osteoporosis, you would expect orthopedic surgeons, who treat broken bones, to be more alert to bone disease. Not so, says Dr. Bilezikian. "A patient with any kind of bone fracture should alert the orthopedist to the need for an evaluation for osteoporosis. Yet we get relatively few referrals a year from our orthopedic surgeons here at Columbia–Presbyterian Medical Center."

The NOF regards physician education as a top priority, says Dr. Lindsay. "It's a matter of getting physicians to the point where, for example, recommending a bone-density test for a 55-year-old woman whose mother just broke her hip becomes automatic."

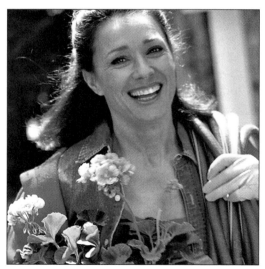

Check Those Bones!

If you have osteoporosis, you're not going to feel your bones weakening. In fact, you may not know that you have it until a bone fractures. That's why it's called the silent disease.

But a bone-density test can mean catching osteoporosis before a debilitating hip or spinal fracture occurs and learning when preventive treatment will be the most effective.

Bone loss is progressive, so detecting someone who is at risk for fractures long before they have osteoporosis is crucial.

Debbie Reynolds Takes On Osteoporosis

Debbie Reynolds, actress, singer, and dancer, is still going strong at age 68. She wishes she could say the same about her bones.

Two years ago, she was diagnosed with osteoporosis. "I was amazed, since I've been exercising and dancing for more than 50 years," says Reynolds, who has delighted audiences in everything from *Singing in the Rain* to *Mother*.

But her grandmother had it, making her a prime candidate for the disease. Today, she's spokeswoman for a national educational campaign called "Stay Strong! Test Your Bone Strength."

"I want to be part of getting the word out to women that having your bones tested is equally as important as getting your mammogram," says Reynolds.

Reynolds learned firsthand just how devastating this disease can be. "My grandmother suffered with osteoporosis, only it didn't have a name back in the 1940s and 1950s. She was very stooped over. My mother sewed her clothes and made them longer in the neck to fit the curve. I pray that with proper guidance from my doctor, I will not have this condition. I don't want the same thing happening to me.

"Women need to talk to their doctors about their risk for osteoporosis and about getting a bone-density test, which is easy and painless," she says. "We can prevent fractures with treatment now, so there's no reason that women shouldn't take steps to stop bone loss and its terrifying effects."

Now that Reynolds knows that her bones are more vulnerable, she's taking steps to play it safe. She has started taking bone-building medication and swims, does yoga, and uses light weights for strengthening her muscles. "This diagnosis has made me more cautious," she adds. "I walk instead of run up and down the steps. I will continue performing, but my show is as much stress as I'm going to put on my body. I want my life to be of quality, not spent in a wheelchair."

Do You Know the Risk Factors for Osteoporosis?

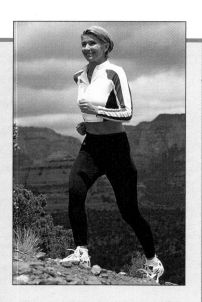

The majority of women in a *Prevention* magazine osteoporosis survey—70 percent—knew that a diet low in calcium put them at risk for developing osteoporosis, and 53 percent knew that not exercising enough increased their risk as well.

But only 38 percent of women 50 and older knew that menopause itself increases the risk—perhaps by as much as 50 percent—because of the loss of estrogen. Here is a list of the major risk factors.

1. A personal history of bone fracture as an adult
2. A history of fractures in a first-degree relative (mother, grandmother, sister)
3. Current cigarette smoking
4. A slender build (less than 127 pounds for an average-size woman)
5. Use of steroid medications
6. Estrogen deficiency caused by early menopause or the removal of ovaries
7. Any loss of menstrual periods for 6 months or more (with the exception of pregnancy)
8. Heavy alcohol consumption
9. Lack of physical activity
10. Lifelong diet low in calcium, vitamin D, or other key nutrients

"Bone loss is progressive, so detecting someone who is at risk for fractures long before they have osteoporosis is crucial," says Sandra C. Raymond, executive director of the National Osteoporosis Foundation.

"Bone-density tests are accurate at predicting the risk of osteoporotic fracture, yet they are underutilized," says Raymond. Only 7 percent of people with osteoporosis have been diagnosed. And according to our survey, only 21 percent of women 50 and older say that a doctor has recommended that they have the test.

Tell your doctor that you want to be tested if you fit into one or more of the following categories.

• A woman age 65 or older
• A postmenopausal woman under age 65 with one or more risk factors for osteoporosis (other than menopause)
• A postmenopausal woman who has had a fracture
• A woman who is considering treatment for osteoporosis

• A woman who has been on estrogen-replacement therapy for prolonged periods

Even women in their thirties and forties who haven't yet reached menopause should have a bone-density test if they don't follow a bone-healthy lifestyle or have one or more risk factors for osteoporosis.

The best type of bone-density test to get is a DEXA (or DXA). This test measures bone at both the hip and spine, where it matters the most. DEXA can detect bone loss at a very early stage, which enables you to take action before severe loss sets in. If this test isn't offered in your area, here is a list of some other options to consider.

• QCT (quantitative computed tomography) of the spine
• US (ultrasound) of the heel
• p-DEXA of the forearm
• PIXI (peripheral instantaneous x-ray image) of the heel and forearm
• SXA (single energy x-ray absorptiometry) of the heel and forearm
• AccuDEXA of the middle finger

Good Stuff for Your Bones

You know that calcium helps fight osteoporosis. But did you know that at least four other vitamins and minerals might play supporting roles? What's troubling is that the average woman's diet is running low in every single one of these support nutrients.

Nutrient	Your Daily Goal	What the Average Woman Gets	Why Bones Love It	Best Food Sources
Vitamin D	400 IU up to age 50; 800 IU age 50 plus	More than half get too little, a 1998 study suggests.	Absorbs calcium from your diet; helps deposit calcium in bone.	Milk and some fortified breakfast cereals; take a multi-vitamin for insurance
Vitamin K	100 mcg may be best for bones.	65 mcg	"Switches on" a bone-building protein called osteocalcin	Spinach, Brussels sprouts, broccoli, asparagus, cabbage, coleslaw, collard greens
Magnesium	400 mg	228 mg	Makes up part of bone; needed to keep blood calcium levels normal	Nuts, dried beans, crabmeat, spinach, wheat germ, wheat bran, chocolate
Potassium	3,500 mg	2,237 mg	May buffer acid in blood so calcium isn't pulled from bones	Fruits and vegetables, lobster, salmon, milk, yogurt

Chapter 18

Control Diabetes Naturally with Herbs

These down-to-earth remedies help balance your blood sugar.

D iabetes has been called the disease of civilization. Our basic nutritional needs have not evolved in the past 100,000 years, but our palates have, and diabetes is closely related to diet.

While our ancient ancestors may have dined on fruits and vegeta-

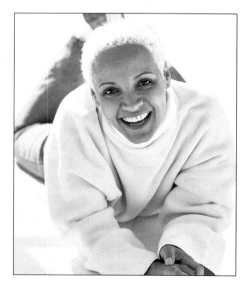

bles, nuts and seeds, and an occasional kill of wild game, we're more partial to double cheeseburgers with a side of fries. Wash that down with a large soda, and you have the recipe for diabetes. Our civilized appetite for foods that are high in sugar and fat can cause metabolic changes that result in chronically high blood sugar, or diabetes. Like the complex civilization in which we live, this pervasive disease is not easily understood or easily treated.

A Complex Disease Explained

To start with the basics, the cells in our bodies need energy to function. They get that energy from glucose, also called blood sugar, which is absorbed when we eat carbohydrates. As the level of glucose builds in your bloodstream, your body secretes a hormone called insulin. Like a key unlocking a door, insulin unleashes the stored energy in the blood and allows it to enter the cells.

There are two main types of diabetes. In both, glucose fails to enter the cells and accumulates in the blood. Over the long term, elevated blood sugar levels can damage the eyes, kidneys, blood vessels, and nerves. Because bacteria thrive on the glucose-rich blood and urine, people with untreated diabetes are also more prone to urinary tract infections.

In type 1, or insulin-dependent diabetes, the pancreas loses its ability to produce insulin. Without that hormone, the glucose absorbed from food remains in the blood, even though the cells are starved for energy. A person with this type of diabetes must inject insulin regularly to help their cells absorb glucose.

About 90 to 95 percent of all people with diabetes have type 2, or non-insulin-dependent, diabetes. With this type, your body may produce enough insulin in the early stages of the condition, but in time, your cells aren't able to respond

Stevia: Sweeter Than Sugar

With virtually no calories and no effect on blood sugar levels, stevia is a safe herbal alternative to sugar or artificial sweeteners, says C. Leigh Broadhurst, Ph.D., a nutrition consultant and herbal researcher based in Clovery, Maryland, and a diabetes researcher with the USDA Human Nutrition Research Center in Beltsville. You won't find it next to aspartame or saccharin in your grocery store, though. Because of Food and Drug Administration restrictions, it is sold only as a dietary supplement.

Derived from the leaves of the wild shrub *Stevia rebaudiana*, which grows in the mountains of Paraguay, stevia is estimated to be 150 to 400 times sweeter than sugar. You need to use just a drop or a pinch, not a spoonful.

Dr. Broadhurst recommends using stevia extract, which is sold by the ounce in health food stores as a liquid or white powder, but remember to use only a small amount. To get accustomed to the taste, Dr. Broadhurst suggests blending it with sugar to get the level of sweetness you want with less sugar.

Finely powdered, dried stevia leaf is also sold in bulk or packaged like tea bags. The distinctive flavor of the greenish powder is similar to that of licorice and blends well with cinnamon and ginger.

to it, and they become insulin-resistant. Blood sugar levels rise, but the energy-starved cells are unable to tap into their fuel supply, so they trigger the body to produce more insulin. When repeated continuously, this process eventually overworks and depletes the supply of special insulin-creating cells in the pancreas until they can no longer function. In an endless merry-go-round of symptoms, the disease perpetuates itself.

Herbs Shown to Help

While both types of diabetes are serious diseases that require a doctor's care, you can use herbs to help regulate your blood sugar, says Robert Rountree, M.D., a holistic physician at the Helios Health Center in Boulder, Colorado.

Herbs aren't substitutes for the fundamental changes in diet and lifestyle that you need to make in order to control your diabetes. You still have to eat right, control your weight, and exercise regularly, says Nancy Welliver, N.D., director of the Institute of Medical Herbalism in Calistoga, California. Medicinal herbs can complement those efforts by lowering blood sugar levels, helping your body use insulin effectively, and protecting you from diabetes-related damage.

It's crucial for people with diabetes to take a daily multivitamin supplement to correct any nutritional deficiencies and to take at least 200 micrograms of chromium daily, says Dr. Welliver. Studies of people with diabetes have shown that supplementing the diet with this trace mineral can regulate blood sugar levels, improve glucose tolerance, and help maintain proper insulin levels. If you have diabetes, don't exceed 400 to 600 micrograms of chromium a day, and be sure

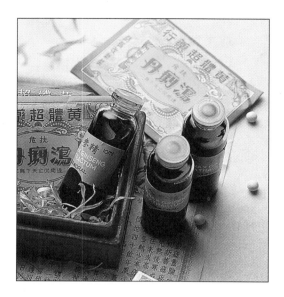

Ginseng can help **stabilize blood sugar levels** if you have type 2 diabetes.

to have your doctor carefully monitor your blood sugar levels.

It's safest to work with a practitioner trained in the use of herbs and other supplements who can develop a protocol specifically for you. Many nutrients and herbs can affect drug doses and regulation. Here's an idea of the types of herbs you can use to manage this complex problem.

Asian Ginseng (*Panax ginseng*)

Known as a feel-good herb that boosts vitality, ginseng can help stabilize blood sugar levels if you have type 2 diabetes, says C. Leigh Broadhurst, Ph.D., a nutrition consultant and herbal researcher based in Clovery, Maryland, and a diabetes researcher with the USDA Human Nutrition Research Center in Beltsville. Take a daily dose of 200 milligrams in capsule form. Asian ginseng may cause irritability if taken with caffeine or other stimulants, and it shouldn't be taken if you have high blood pressure.

For centuries, practitioners of Traditional Chinese Medicine have used ginseng to treat diabetes. Now, Western practitioners are catching on. In a study in Finland, researchers found that a daily dose of 200 milligrams of ginseng for 8 weeks improved mood, diet, and activity, which reduced weight and helped lower blood sugar levels.

Bilberry (*Vaccinium myrtillus*)

Since 1945, French doctors have used bilberry to prevent diabetic retinopathy. While the leaves of this European version of the blueberry lower

---

Cut Diabetes Risk in Half

Studies have already suggested a link between increased physical activity and decreased chances for developing type 2 diabetes. Exercise of any kind trims your odds by improving your body's sensitivity to insulin. For diabetics, this hormone may either be in low supply or difficult for the body to use.

Activity also helps control cholesterol, weight, and blood pressure, which further guards you from adult-onset diabetes.

But what experts hadn't understood was how powerfully protective a fast-paced stroll could be, until Harvard University researchers examined the exercise habits of more than 70,000 women. Here's what their findings suggest.

Get your daily 40. Lead researcher Frank B. Hu, M.D., assistant professor of nutrition at the Harvard School of Public Health, says that even in people with risk factors such as added pounds, high cholesterol, high blood pressure, or a family history of diabetes, hitting the pavement for a brisk 40-minute walk every day dropped risk a significant 40 percent.

Even better, walk for an hour. The study findings suggest that a little more walking may be even more protective. A fast-paced 60-minute walk every day could cut the risk in half, Dr. Hu says.

Keep it brisk, but comfortable. The most beneficial speed? Three miles an hour—a comfortable 20 minutes per mile. Walking at a normal, average pace of 2 to 2½ miles per hour reduced risk by 20 to 30 percent.

Not into walking? By all means, try something else. Other vigorous activities, from swimming laps to tennis to bicycling, can also lower your diabetes risk.

blood sugar levels, the flavonoid-rich fruit provides potent antioxidant effects that improve the circulation of blood in the eyes for those with both types of diabetes, says Dr. Welliver. Take 80 milligrams of extract twice a day to reduce the risk of retinopathy.

Bitter Melon (*Momordica charantia*)

Because it works on so many levels, bitter melon is the best herb to start with to help control diabetes and its complications, says Dr. Welliver. This Asian food has been used traditionally as a remedy for diabetes. Eating bitter melon increases the insulin-secreting cells in the pancreas, called beta cells. It is thought to help regulate blood sugar levels by slowing the absorption of glucose. According to Dr. Welliver, studies suggest that bitter melon is most effective for type 2 diabetes and possibly early type 1.

To help regulate your blood sugar levels, drink 2 ounces of bitter melon juice twice a day.

Cultivated throughout the tropical regions of the world, bitter melon is used as an anti-diabetes remedy in China, India, Sri Lanka, and the West Indies. It's available in the United States at Asian markets. You can make the juice by running the fruit through a juicer or by pureeing it in a blender with a little water until it is thin enough to drink. You can take bitter melon indefinitely at these dosages. Looking farther down the road, a daily shot of bitter melon juice may reduce your risk of developing diabetic retinopathy, a complication of diabetes caused by damage to blood vessels of the retina, says Dr. Welliver.

Cinnamon (*Cinnamomum zeylanicum*)

Cinnamon contains a phytochemical that helps those with both type 1 and type 2 diabetes utilize blood sugar, says Dr. Broadhurst. In the past 10 years, researchers at the USDA Beltsville Nutrient Requirements and Functions Laboratory in Maryland have tested 60 other medicinal and food plants looking for the same anti-diabetes effect.

"Nothing has come close to the consistently excellent results of cinnamon," says Dr. Broadhurst. "Since the first report on cinnamon, hundreds of people have contacted the laboratory to

While diabetes is a serious disease that requires a doctor's care, you can **use herbs to help regulate your blood sugar**.

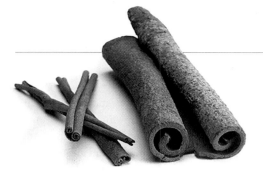

Hundreds of people say cinnamon helped **reduce their medication dosages**.

say how cinnamon has helped them reduce their insulin or medication dosages."

To help your body utilize blood sugar naturally, drink 1 quart of cinnamon water every day. Sounds like a lot, doesn't it? One way to make sure you get the recommended dosage is to make up a batch of this pleasant-tasting beverage and substitute it for part of your daily water intake. Add 3 tablespoons of cinnamon and 2 teaspoons of baking soda to 1 quart of boiling water. Reduce the temperature and simmer for 20 minutes, then strain the mixture and store it in the refrigerator.

The flavor and quality of cinnamon vary according to the quality of its volatile oils. Since the active ingredient is a water-based chemical, it doesn't matter what type you use to make this tea, says Dr. Broadhurst. It will be just as effective with a cheaper, less aromatic spice. If you find that cinnamon helps you, you can use it regularly.

Flaxseed (*Linum usitatissimum*)

Ground flaxseed is one of nature's richest sources of soluble fiber. It improves your body's ability to metabolize blood sugar in type 1 or type 2 diabetes, explains Dr. Broadhurst.

Eat 2 tablespoons daily. Stir it into a glass of water or sprinkle it on your cereal. Your daily allotment can also be added to blender drinks, oatmeal, or baked goods on a regular basis, she says. No matter how you choose to incorporate it into your diet, be sure to drink at least 8 ounces of water when you take it. And don't take flaxseed at all if you have a bowel obstruction.

Ginkgo (*Ginkgo biloba*)

Known for its ability to improve memory, ginkgo can also improve circulation and help reduce your risk of complications such as eye problems or ulcers on your hands and feet, says Dr.

HOLLYWOOD HEALTH
Miss America Reigns Over Diabetes

"When I first was diagnosed with diabetes, I thought I was dying," recalls former Miss America Nicole Johnson, who has type 1 diabetes. "But once I better educated myself about the disease, I learned that I could control it," she says. Although a diagnosis of type 1 or 2 diabetes will necessitate some lifestyle changes, it is possible to live a happy, healthy life with the disease.

Welliver. Native to China, the ginkgo tree is thought to be the oldest tree on the planet, originating more than 190 million years ago. Take 80 milligrams of the concentrated extract in capsule form three times a day.

Ginkgo has the potential to interact with prescription drugs. Do not use it with antide-pressant MAO inhibitor drugs such as phenelzine sulfate (Nardil) or tranylcypromine (Parnate), aspirin or other nonsteroidal anti-inflammatory medications, or blood-thinning medications such as warfarin (Coumadin). And don't exceed the recommended dosage, as dosages higher than 240 milligrams of the concentrated extract can

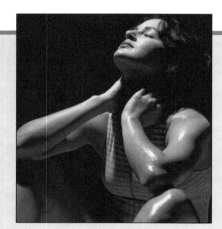

Harness the Newest Ally against Diabetes: Your Mind

Take a deep breath. Let your muscles go limp. A small study of 18 people with diabetes suggests that simple relaxation exercises such as these can reduce blood sugar levels by 9 to 12 percent.

But relaxation techniques may be most effective as allies for blood sugar control if you're already tuned in to your state of mind, says lead study author Angele McGrady, Ph.D., professor of psychology and physiology at the Medical College of Ohio in Toledo. They didn't appear to help those who were depressed or anxious. Here's what you can do.

Relax and reflect in solitude. Sharpen self-awareness and practice relaxation with regular time alone, Dr. McGrady suggests. Start with a minute or two of deep breathing, then spend 10 to 15 minutes progressively relaxing your body. Start with your feet, and work your way up. Tell yourself that the muscles in each body part are heavy, warm, and loose.

Practice prevention. Reduce bouts of anxiety by avoiding stimulants such as caffeine, maintaining a healthy diet, and exercising regularly. Spend time with friends who boost your spirits.

Target your triggers. Are you facing a situation that has you worked up or has made you feel down in the past? Give yourself something positive to focus on by planning, in advance, an activity, outing, or project that you know short-circuits depression or anxiety.

cause dermatitis, diarrhea, and vomiting.

Gurmur (*Gymnema sylvestre*)

The leaves of this climbing vine have been used in traditional Ayurvedic medicine as a treatment for diabetes, says Dr. Welliver. "It seems to enhance the production of insulin, possibly through the regeneration of beta cells of the pancreas," she says. That would make it appropriate for people with type 2 diabetes and even those with early type 1. Take 400 milligrams in capsule form twice a day.

Another added benefit: Gurmur may help curb your sweet tooth. "It has the unusual property of blocking sugary taste. Since the sweet satisfaction isn't as pronounced, you aren't as tempted to consume large amounts of it," according to Dr. Welliver. The herb is safe to use on a regular basis, she says.

1-MINUTE FAT BURNER

Trick your taste-buds. Sucking on a sugar-free menthol-eucalyptus cough drop can stop cravings instantly.

Prickly Pear (*Opuntia ficusindica*)

The soluble fiber in this traditional Latin American food slows the absorption of glucose from the intestines, says Dr. Welliver. Studies began on the anti-diabetes activity of prickly pear (also known as Nopal cactus) in the 1920s. Researchers now theorize that it may improve the effectiveness of available insulin in people with type 2 diabetes by stimulating glucose to move from the bloodstream into body cells.

Eat 1 cup of prickly pear a day. "You have to eat the real thing," cautions Dr. Welliver. "All the studies showed that using capsules had no effect."

Don't worry if you don't live in the desert, though. Canned prickly pear is available in health food stores and some grocery stores, and it's safe to enjoy on an ongoing basis.

Chapter 19

Cancer Tests That Are Worth Your Life

These are lifesaving tests your insurance may not cover—but you should.

Nearly 1 in 30 Americans alive today has been diagnosed with cancer. That's more than 8 million of us—enough to form a Rockettes-style chorus line reaching one-third of the way around the Earth. For more than half of those, it's been 5 or more years since their diagnosis.

That's pretty impressive, particularly when you consider that just one or two generations ago, the odds of surviving cancer were mighty slim. Improved treatment has helped, but so have earlier diagnosis and cancer screening.

"With screenings that can detect certain cancers early, when they're most treatable, we can significantly increase a person's chances of surviving those cancers," says Therese Bevers, M.D., medical director of clinical

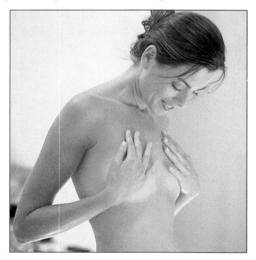

cancer prevention at the University of Texas M.D. Anderson Cancer Center in Houston. Some tests can even detect certain precancerous conditions, so they can be monitored and treated before they ever progress to cancer.

Will Your Insurance Cover It?

Health insurance plans that cover preventive care often cover some, if not all, of the cost of screening tests. But even if your plan doesn't cover a particular test, it may be worth getting it and paying for it yourself.

Which tests should you consider shelling out for? That depends on your circumstances—how old you are, whether certain forms of cancer run in your family, whether you smoked during a profligate youth—and is something to hash out with your physician, says Dr. Bevers. Here, to get you started, is a list of less frequently covered screening tests recommended by leading cancer experts.

Colon Cancer: Genetic Testing

Genetic tests can detect mutations linked to two forms of colon cancer, familial polyposis and hereditary nonpolyposis colon cancer (HNPCC).

If one of your parents had familial polyposis, you should consider paying for genetic coun-

> # 1-MINUTE
> ## FAT BURNER
>
> **Skip "light" foods. The weight of a food—not just the fat and calories—is what fills you up. Eat less and still feel satisfied with low-calorie heavy-weights such as oranges, strawberries, grapefruit, cantaloupe, cooked spinach, collard greens, and broccoli. Plus, the fiber helps protect against cancer.**

seling and these one-time tests, says Harold Frucht, M.D., director of gastroenterology at Fox Chase Cancer Center in Philadelphia. Ditto if you have three relatives with HNPCC-associated tumors. If you test positive for one of the mutations, you should have a colonoscopy, in which a physician uses a lighted flexible scope to check inside your colon, every 1 to 2 years. The colonoscopy can detect areas with precancerous changes in your colon so that physicians can remove them before they become cancerous.

Note: Unlike the genetic tests, the colonoscopy should be covered by your insurance.

Cost: $750 to $2,000

Endometrial and Ovarian Cancers: Biopsy, Ultrasound, and CA-125 Testing

Endometrial biopsy and an alternative exam, transvaginal ultrasound, can help to detect endometrial cancer. But both are controversial because it's not yet clear if they can detect the cancer earlier than it would be diagnosed if symptoms such as abnormal vaginal bleeding were present, explains Dr. Bevers.

Women at high risk for endometrial cancer—a group that includes women who have taken or are currently taking tamoxifen (Nolvadex), a drug for treatment or prevention of breast cancer, and women with an inherited form of colon cancer called hereditary nonpolyposis colon cancer

(HNPCC)—should discuss the pros and cons of endometrial biopsy or transvaginal ultrasound with their doctors, says Dr. Bevers.

When transvaginal ultrasound is combined with the CA-125 blood test, it may also help diagnose ovarian cancer. The CA-125 test measures levels of a protein called glycoprotein OC125, which is produced by cancer cells. But this test is controversial too, in part because it can yield false-negative results, giving the all-clear even when there's really an increased cancer risk, says Matthew Boente, M.D., chief of gynecologic oncology at Fox Chase Cancer Center in Philadelphia.

To further muddle matters, the CA-125 test can also net false-positive results, particularly in premenopausal patients. That's why the best approach is to combine an ultrasound with CA-125 testing when checking for ovarian cancer.

Women with BRCA1 and BRCA2 mutations—genetic errors that have been linked to ovarian, breast, and some other types of cancer—should consider getting these tests twice yearly. If ovarian cancer runs in your family, you should also consider getting them every 6 months, recommends Mary Daly, M.D., Ph.D., director of family risk assessment programs at Fox Chase Cancer Center in Philadelphia.

At least one study has shown that regular testing may be promising for detecting early-stage ovarian cancer.

Get This Follow-Up Test

A recent study of more than 24,000 women and men over age 65 found that just 1 in 3 people with an increased risk of colon cancer got the follow-up test that saves lives.

Chalk it up to squeamishness—or perhaps to doctor oversight, according to lead study author Jon D. Lurie, M.D., assistant professor of medicine at Dartmouth Hitchcock Medical Center in Lebanon, New Hampshire. Everyone in the study had a fecal occult blood test (FOBT), which checks for blood in the stool—a warning flag that cancer might be present. But of the 2,245 people with positive FOBTs, only 34 percent took a follow-up test.

Early detection is key. Just 4 percent of positive FOBTs are cancerous, but doctors can't tell unless they can get a closer look with either a sigmoidoscopy (with a barium enema) or a colonoscopy. Both of these use a flexible, lighted tube with a camera on one end that is inserted into the colon.

Light sedation makes these follow-ups more comfortable. Though they can sound scary, the payoff is well worth it. Both can detect early signs of cancer, and with early detection, there is a high cure rate.

Cost: Roughly $250 for endometrial biopsy, and an additional $100 to $200 for the pathologist's fee; about $200 for transvaginal ultrasound alone; and roughly $250 to $500 for a transvaginal ultrasound and CA-125 blood test

Breast Cancer: Early Mammography

Insurance plans often cover annual mammograms for women age 40 and older. But if two or more of your close relatives have had breast cancer—particularly if they were diagnosed before their fortieth birthdays—it's a good idea to start getting annual mammograms before you celebrate yours.

Your insurer may not cover early mammograms even if you have a family history of the disease, says Dr. Daly. If that's the case, consider paying out-of-pocket.

Cost: $75 to $150

Breast Cancer: Annual Clinical Breast Exam

A professional version of the self-exam every woman should practice monthly (you do, don't you?), a clinical breast exam (CBE) helps physicians interpret your mammogram. The exam can also pick up tumors that don't show up in a mammogram, says Dr. Bevers.

Lower Your Breast Cancer Risk by Half

Postmenopausal women may be able to cut their risk of breast cancer in half by being active. When researchers followed 1,806 women (average age 75) for 11 years, they found that those who were moderately active (walking, gardening, or doing housework several times a week) had a 50 percent lower risk of breast cancer compared to sedentary women. The women who did vigorous activity—swimming, running, or playing tennis at least once a week—were 80 percent less likely to develop the disease.

"Getting active—and that can mean starting to walk regularly—or staying active appears to be important in the elderly," says study author James R. Cerhan, M.D., Ph.D., of the Mayo Clinic, in Rochester, Minnesota. Most of the research on the role that physical activity plays in the development of breast cancer has involved younger women. But this new study suggests that it's never too late.

"Most breast cancer authorities would say a CBE needs to be done as close to an annual mammogram as possible," Dr. Bevers says. Some insurers such as Medicare, however, pay the tab for CBEs only once every 3 years in conjunction with a pelvic exam and Pap test. If yours is among them, it's probably worth covering the tab for an annual CBE yourself.

Cost: $45 to $55. Keep in mind: Even if your insurance doesn't cover annual CBEs, you may not always have to pay out-of-pocket.

Finding Freebies

If your health insurance plan doesn't cover a particular cancer screening test, you may still be able to get it without pulling out your checkbook.

Research centers studying experimental screening exams may offer them at no charge to volunteers who meet their study criteria, explains Mary Daly, M.D., Ph.D., director of family risk assessment programs at Philadelphia's Fox Chase Cancer Center.

To find a nearby center that may be offering free experimental screening tests or clinical trials, call the National Cancer Institute at (800) 4-CANCER (422-6237). The NCI may also be able to refer people who meet certain eligibility requirements to programs that provide low-cost mammograms and Pap tests.

Though some insurers won't cover an annual CBE for screening purposes, many will cover the test if it's done for diagnostic purposes: to determine the cause of breast pain, or some other disconcerting symptom.

Genetic Mutation Cancers: Genetic Counseling

In a genetic counseling session, a counselor analyzes your family's health history—everything from your Uncle Harry's "spells" to your grandpa's prostate problems—to determine whether you're likely to have inherited a genetic glitch such as the BRCA1 or BRCA2 mutation. If the answer is yes, the counselor will recommend genetic testing with a blood test. And if the tests are positive, she may recommend further tests, more frequent screening, and preventive measures to increase your odds of beating cancer.

Even if genetic testing shows that you're free and clear of the nefarious mutations that scientists have already linked to the disease, you may have inherited a susceptibility to cancer that involves as-yet-undiscovered mutations. Genetic counseling can help identify your vulnerabilities.

While many insurers cover genetic testing for mutations such as BRCA1 and BRCA2, they may not pay for counseling, say Dr. Daly and Dr. Bevers. If yours doesn't, and you're interested in genetic testing, they agree that you should consider paying out-of-pocket for counseling first.

Cost: About $200

Lung Cancer: Low-Dose CAT Scan Screening

Lung cancer, which kills more Americans than any other kind of cancer, usually isn't diagnosed until it's too far gone to treat. That's because

Screening Tests: You're Probably Covered

The following American Cancer Society–endorsed screening tests, designed to detect relatively common cancers, are at least partly covered by Medicare and a good number of private insurance plans that emphasize preventive care.

Note: Since private plans vary considerably, check with your insurer to find out what yours covers.

Breast Cancer
Women age 40 and older should get an annual mammogram and clinical breast exam (CBE) and should do monthly breast self-exams (BSE). Women ages 20 to 39 should get a CBE every 3 years and do a BSE monthly.

Coverage: Medicare and many insurers cover annual mammograms in part or full for beneficiaries who are age 40 and older.

Colon and Rectal Cancer
Women age 50 and older should follow one of these examination schedules.
- A fecal occult blood test (FOBT) every year and both a flexible sigmoid-oscopy and digital rectal exam (DRE) every 5 years
- A colonoscopy and DRE every 10 years
- A double-contrast barium enema and a DRE every 5 to 10 years

Coverage: Medicare and many plans that emphasize preventive care cover the fecal occult, sigmoidoscopy, colonoscopy, and barium enema tests for beneficiaries age 50 and older.

Cervical Cancer
Women age 18 and older and all women who are or have been sexually active should get an annual Pap test and pelvic exam.

Note: If you've had three or more consecutive normal Pap tests, your physician may recommend less frequent Pap tests.

Coverage: Medicare and most health plans cover the Pap test, although Medicare restricts it to once every 3 years in most cases.

chest x-rays and other medical tests aren't sensitive enough to detect most lung tumors when they're small enough to be cured.

A recent study, however, suggests that annual low-dose CAT scans may do the trick, detecting tumors considerably earlier, when they're treatable.

More sensitive than x-rays, low-dose CAT

scans could greatly improve the odds of surviving lung cancer, says the study's lead author, Claudia I. Henschke, M.D., head of the division of chest imaging at Weill Medical College of Cornell University in New York City.

If you're 60 or older and a smoker, or a former smoker, Dr. Henschke suggests that you consider getting a lung CAT scan annually, though the test usually isn't covered by insurance. Initial scans tend to have high false-positive rates, turning up benign as well as cancerous tumors. Subsequent scans are more accurate because the radiologist is looking only for changes since the previous scan.

Make sure that you see an experienced chest radiologist who is best able to distinguish benign from cancerous growths, adds study coauthor David Naidich, M.D., director of thoracic imaging at New York University Medical Center in New York City.

Cost: About $300

Skin Cancer: Total-Body Skin Examination and Photography

During a total-body skin exam, a physician, usually a dermatologist, checks your birthday suit for suspicious moles and related growths and for changes in these growths since your last visit. These can be signs of precancer or cancer.

Few insurers cover a total-body skin exam, but it's a worthwhile investment if you run a higher-than-average risk of skin cancer, says Jean-Claude Bystryn, M.D., director of the melanoma program at the Kaplan Comprehensive Cancer Center in New York City. People at highest risk—those who've already had the form of skin cancer called melanoma—should get screened several times a year.

If someone in your family has had melanoma and you have additional risk factors—you have spent more time in the sun than George Hamilton, have had lots of sunburns, have fair skin or many moles—get screened twice a year. If skin cancer runs in your family, but you have no other risk factors, a once-a-year check should do, Dr. Bystryn says.

Speaking of moles: If you really have a lot of them, total-body photographs may also be worth investing in, Dr. Bystryn adds. They're just what they sound like: photographs of your entire body, documenting where your skin growths are and what they look like, so your physician can more accurately track changes.

Cost: From $50 to $200 for a total-body skin exam; about $300 for total-body photography

Liver Cancer: Liver Ultrasound

If you have chronic hepatitis B or C, which substantially raises your risk of cancer, your insurance usually covers a semiannual liver cancer screening test, called the alpha-fetal protein (AFP) test. Elevated AFP levels can be a warning sign of liver cancer. If the test shows elevated AFP levels, doctors follow it with an ultrasound for a better picture of what's happening down in the depths of your liver, explains Thomas London, M.D., a liver cancer specialist at Fox Chase Cancer Center in Philadelphia.

Many physicians recommend doing the ultrasound every 2 to 3 months if AFP levels stay elevated. But not all insurers cover such frequent ultrasound testing, Dr. London says. If you have chronic hepatitis B or C and your AFP levels remain elevated, you may want to get an ultrasound test every 2 months, even if you have to pay part of the cost, he says.

Cost: About $425

LIFESTYLE RESTYLE

She Found the Support She Needed

At age 29, Olivia Williamson found out she had high blood pressure. Her doctor told her that unless she did something about it, she could be on drugs for the rest of her life.

Williamson knew what that "something" was. After all, she weighed 240 pounds. "I had no choice but to slim down. Having high blood pressure really scared me," she says.

It's not that she hadn't tried before; diet and exercise regimens were no strangers to Williamson. But she could never stick with them on her own. This time, she decided, she'd enlist help.

Luckily for Williamson, her employer, Stanford University, offers a 6-week healthy-weight-management class through the school's medical center. Once the class is over, students can attend weekly support-group meetings for up to 4 months. Williamson signed on.

For the first 10 weeks, she diligently followed the directions of the class instructor, cutting back on fat, eating less in one sitting, and exercising moderately. But she didn't lose a single pound. Was she frustrated? You bet. But the support group kept Williamson going.

In the group, she met people who were facing the exact same challenges she was. It was a perfect forum for exchanging advice on what works and what doesn't, for unloading frustrations, and for celebrating victories. "Just being able to tell the group, 'I'm doing it; I'm sticking with it' made me feel better," says Williamson, of Mountain View, California. "It allowed me to settle into the healthier habits that I was learning." She enjoyed the group so much that when her weight-management course ended, she joined an e-mail diet-support network she found through Stanford.

Within a year, Williamson lost 45 pounds, and her blood pressure returned to a healthy level. As a bonus, she had more energy than ever before, which encouraged her to stay active in her daily life. "When I went on a sightseeing trip to Europe in 1999, I was able to climb all 340 steps to the top of Notre Dame Cathedral," she says. "I wouldn't have been able to do that before!"

To locate a support group near you, start by calling local hospitals and churches. Look in the blue pages of your phone book, under Self-Help Support Groups. Or check whether your employer keeps a list of local resources.

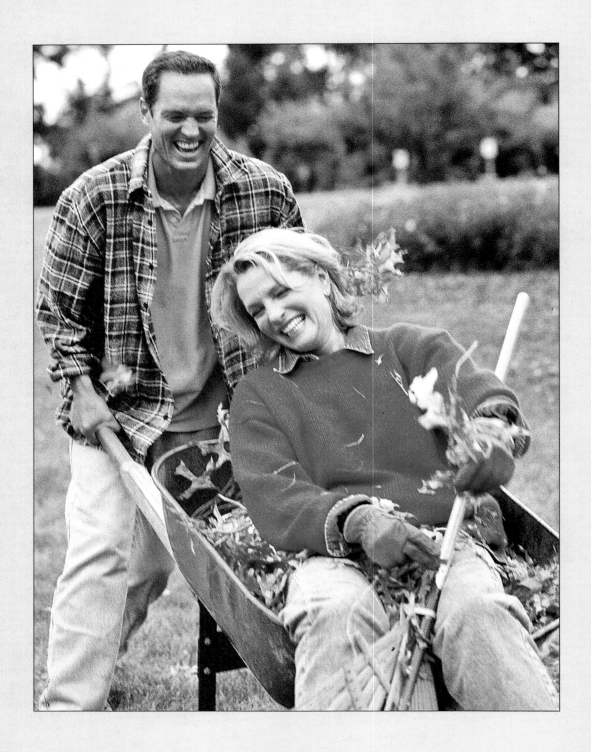

Part Five

Relax Your Mind, Rejuvenate Your Soul

Chapter 20

Learn to Breathe "Right"

Try it to lower blood pressure, increase stamina, enhance mood, and boost libido.

We breathe about 20,000 times a day—that's more than 500 million breaths in a lifetime—yet experts say that most of us don't even do it correctly. If we did, we could be healthier.

It's one of the most fundamental aspects of our lives. A human can survive without food for more than 2 months and without water for

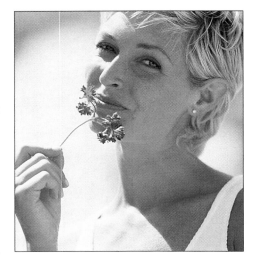

about a week, but after 4 minutes without breathing, brain damage begins, followed quickly by death.

Breathing does far more than just keep us alive. Research has shown that it delivers a cornucopia of health benefits, among them reduced tension, increased stamina and endurance, improved athletic performance, better digestion, lowered high blood pressure, less fatigue, weight loss, improved sleep, less constipation, enhanced memory and mood, increased libido, and improved work efficiency. More than simply being the flow of air into and out of our lungs, breathing is, in fact, a tool that can improve life on every level.

‖ Breathe
‖ like a Baby

The first step you need to take is to become more aware of your breathing.

"Most of us do what I call upside-down breathing," says Gay Hendricks, Ph.D., president of the Hendricks Institute in Santa Barbara, California, and author of *Conscious Breathing: Breathwork for Health, Stress Release, and Personal Mastery*. He points out that we tighten our stomach muscles as we inhale, filling our upper chests with air, then relax our abdomens on the exhale.

But the experts say that's backward. To see the correct way to breathe, watch babies: Their abdomens rise on the inhale and contract on the exhale. This is called belly, or diaphragmatic, breathing. The key is to fully exhale before inhaling again. Dr. Hendricks says that this form of

Breathwork Glossary

Breathwork is an umbrella term covering a wide variety of techniques. Here are three of the most common ones.

Alternate nostril breathing. This originated with yogic practices but now enjoys wider applications for such things as stress reduction and fighting fatigue. It involves closing one nostril as you forcibly breathe through the other, then switching nostrils. Alternating between the two nostrils reputedly stimulates both hemispheres of the brain: Breathing through the right nostril stimulates your left brain, used for logical, linear thinking; while breathing through the left stimulates your right brain, the seat of creativity and emotions.

Holotropic breathing. Developed by Stanislav Grof, M.D., this technique combines elements from aboriginal traditions, Eastern spirituality, and Western psychology to help people release trapped emotions. Employed in a workshop setting, the method relies on continuous fast, deep breathing and evocative music to help people attain altered states of consciousness.

Transform breathing. Also called full wave breathing, this method was developed by Thomas Goode, N.D., the managing director of the International Breath Institute in Boulder, Colorado. It focuses on not just the diaphragm but also the lower abdomen, solar plexus, and chest. It envisions breath as a metaphor for life, with full and open breathing facilitating a full and open life.

breathing is like an oxygen "cocktail" because of the additional store of the element that it makes available to your body.

Babies may naturally do it right, but as young children become more aware of things they can't physically or emotionally control, everyday stresses cause them to breathe shallowly, not completely emptying their lungs on the exhale. That's part of the fight-or-flight reflex, encoded in us since the Stone Age. As adults, that shallow breathing is reinforced by society encouraging women to suck in their stomachs and men to puff out their chests.

"Most of us spend the entire day in a modified form of the fight-or-flight reflex," says Jeffrey A. Migdow, M.D., a holistic physician in Lennox, Massachusetts, and coauthor of *Breathe In, Breathe Out: Inhale Energy and Exhale Stress by Guiding and Controlling Your Breathing.* "In fact, most people unconsciously hold their breath 80 percent of the time, although optimally, we'd be breathing between 90 and 100 percent of the time."

The resulting increase in adrenaline and heart rate actually causes physical stress; and as many as 90 percent of physician visits are for stress-related disease, estimates Herbert Benson, M.D., head of the Mind/Body Medical Institute at Harvard Medical School and Beth Israel Hospital in Boston. Dr. Benson, a believer in the power of breathing, has shown that a now-fa-

1-MINUTE FAT BURNER

Take a whiff. When you *really* want those fresh-baked cookies, try this: Indulge in the smell for 30 seconds. Then place a small piece on the tip of your tongue for another 30 seconds. Savoring the smell and taste can help you to stop at just one cookie.

mous meditative breath technique, which he dubbed the Relaxation Response, can lower stress and improve health on every level.

Breath and Your Body

Experts have shown that by learning how to breathe correctly and inhale more oxygen, you can help ward off disease and infection. "Most chronic disease is, to some degree, the result of insufficient oxygen," asserts Carl Stough, founder of the Carl Stough Institute of Breathing Coordination in New York City. This lack of oxygen is called hypoxia.

Stough has done extensive research on the diaphragm, the thin, dome-shaped sheet of muscle fiber, similar to a drumhead, that's located between the bottom of the lungs and the top of the abdomen. He points out that while it's capable of moving 12 centimeters during breathing—and 8 centimeters is considered a healthy breath—most people are lucky if they make it move more than 3 centimeters when they breathe.

When there's air left over in your lungs after the end of an exhale (called residual volume), the buildup of carbon dioxide can predispose you to tension, migraine headaches, infections, and, Stough believes, even heart disease and cancer. "There isn't a biopsy of cancer tissue that doesn't show a lack of oxygen," he notes.

Your body is designed to discharge 70 percent of its toxins through breathing, Dr. Hendricks explains. If you don't expel all of the carbon dioxide and other toxins through the breath, he says, 11 other systems must work overtime, setting the stage for a number of illnesses.

His patients report a radical decrease in the number of sick days they take after he teaches them how to breathe properly. "Since I began breathwork in 1974," he adds, "I haven't missed a day of work myself."

Dr. Migdow agrees that the breath is a silent partner in maximizing health. For example, proper breathing can optimize the efficiency of the nervous system. "Since the nervous system has a strong effect on the immune system, breathing correctly can improve immunity," he says. "Warding off a cold is easier when you breathe right, and if you do get sick, it helps you get better faster."

Proper breathing has been credited with helping relieve everything from hot flashes, which can be cut in half, to asthma. Thomas Goode, N.D., managing director of the International Breath Institute in Boulder, Colorado, estimates that 30 percent of all asthma cases are really just shallow breathing.

Breath training can also aid athletes, Dr. Migdow says. Correct breathing relaxes the body and makes muscles more flexible, which increases stamina.

Stough worked with the American athletes as a breathing coach during the 1968 Olympic games in high-altitude Mexico City, teaching them special exercises to retrain their diaphragms to work at optimum efficiency. Subsequently, the United States won more gold medals than any previous American team in the history of the Olympics and were the only ones that didn't require supplemental oxygen.

Dr. Hendricks has also worked with athletes, reporting his most dramatic success with a marathon runner who sliced 30 minutes off her usual 4-hour time after just one breathing lesson.

Other forms of breathwork can help relieve pain or increase energy. The focused hyperventilation techniques used by the Lamaze method of childbirth often lessen the pain of childbirth or at least provide a mental distraction so that it becomes more tolerable.

And you can use short, forced exhalations (the opposite of calming diaphragmatic breathing) whenever you are drowsy or need a pick-me-up. "It makes the fluid around the spine and the brain vibrate," Dr. Migdow explains, "which stimulates the brain and wakes it up."

Warding off a cold is easier when you
breathe right, and if you do get sick,
it helps **you get better faster**.

HealthPoint

Breathe Easier Outside

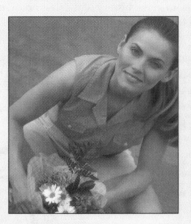

If you think you're safe from air pollution because you don't live in Los Angeles or the Big Apple, think again. Even when you're breathing what you think is fresh mountain air, you may be inhaling enough ozone and other air pollutants to decrease lung function and make breathing more difficult.

In fact, when researchers tested people hiking in the White Mountains in New Hampshire, that's what they found, to a certain degree. Although the average ozone level in the mountains is lower than in much of the country, pollution still has its effect. "Pollutants aren't present only in crowded cities," says Gary Hatch, Ph.D., of the pulmonary toxicology branch of the Environmental Protection Agency in Research Triangle Park, North Carolina.

Inhaling bad air may cause various problems, such as tightness in the chest, coughing, wheezing, and watery eyes. These symptoms can get worse when you exercise. People with asthma, allergies, or respiratory illness; the elderly; and young children are most at risk.

Interestingly, those who continually exercise in high-pollution areas can become accustomed to it over time and have fewer, if any, symptoms, but their lungs may still be negatively affected. Those who exercise in areas with lower pollution levels may not experience symptoms at all but can also have some decline in lung function. Researchers suspect that this decline, which normally oc-

Breath and Your Mind

Optimum breathing improves your mental well-being every bit as much as your physical health. Dr. Migdow regularly teaches patients proper breathing techniques. When they return a month later for a follow-up, they typically report that they've been better able to tolerate tension, he says. "They communicate better with their coworkers and their partners too."

Psychologists use breathwork to help patients through difficult emotional explorations. Shallow breathing can prevent us from feeling safe enough to recognize and release repressed emotional issues, says Dr. Hendricks. "Those

curs as you get older, may speed up and may also be linked with the risk of asthma, respiratory illness, and even lung cancer.

During exercise, you increase your intake of air (and pollutants). You also usually breathe through your mouth rather than your nose. (Your nose filters air better.) Despite the harmful effects that running or walking in polluted urban areas can have, it doesn't mean you have to abandon exercise. Here's how you can get a heart-healthy workout and protect your lungs at the same time.

Get your vitamins. Antioxidants such as vitamins C and E help protect your lungs from damage by pollutants. To get the benefits of these vitamins, eat a diet rich in fruits and vegetables, and take 100 to 500 milligrams of vitamin C and 100 to 400 IU of vitamin E a day.

Watch the weather. Avoid vigorous exercise when air is thick and stagnant. Even a slight breeze can help disperse the concentrations of pollutants in the air, creating better conditions for exercising outdoors. While windy conditions may decrease pollutants, however, they can also stir up pollens and aggravate allergies. In any case, check the air-quality index in your local newspaper or on a TV weather report. If the weather report rates air quality as poor, exercise indoors.

Time it right. Ozone levels peak around noon. If your workout time falls at midday, exercise indoors. Morning and late evening are usually better bets for clean air and outdoor workouts.

Avoid traffic jams. To reduce your exposure to pollution, especially carbon monoxide, avoid exercising on busy streets and during rush hour. Walk, cycle, or run in parks or on side streets.

Whatever your location or weather condition, if you experience tightness in your chest, wheezing, coughing, or difficulty breathing, slow your pace. If that doesn't help, stop exercising. Call a doctor if symptoms persist.

feelings stay lodged in our bodies longer than they need to, setting the stage for a number of physical disorders."

We tend to hold various unexpressed emotions in certain parts of our bodies, Dr. Hendricks explains. When you are "trapped" in an emotion, it's helpful to focus attention on whichever area of your body is tense, while breathing diaphragmatically and visualizing the breath filling the area in question. Typically, your neck, shoulders, and upper back are connected to anger; your throat and upper chest to sadness; and your stomach and intestines to fear.

If you breathe your way through stress, you might also reap the benefit of a sharper mind.

Research by behavioral biologist Robert Sapolsky, Ph.D., of Stanford University shows that the chemicals produced in our bodies when we are stressed damage the region of the brain that is responsible for memory and learning. Reducing stress helps prevent this damage, which in turn helps improve our ability to focus, remember, and learn.

Breath and Your Spirit

Breath can also help you open the door to a richer spiritual life, deepening your connection to a higher power. "Breath truly links mind and body," says Erik Peper, Ph.D., director of the Institute of Holistic Healing Studies at San Fran-

Breathe Your Way out of an Asthma Attack

Can slow inhalation relieve an asthma attack? Maybe, says Paul M. Lehrer, M.D., professor in the department of psychiatry at the University of Medicine and Dentistry of New Jersey Robert Wood Johnson Medical School in Piscataway. He conducted a small study of just 18 men and women and found that breathing and biofeedback may prove to be an effective nondrug approach for helping people decrease asthma symptoms.

Though his study produced its results with the additional aid of a biofeedback machine (which he recommends for best results), Dr. Lehrer believes that practicing the special slow-breathing technique he developed might reduce the frequency of asthma attacks for some people. (*Caution*: Never stop taking your prescribed medications without your doctor's approval.) To try this slow-breathing technique, do the following:

- Breathe at about six breaths a minute, slowly and regularly, for 20 minutes, twice a day.
- Don't inhale too deeply.
- Exhale through pursed lips.
- Breathe from your abdomen.
- If you begin to feel lightheaded, you're hyperventilating. Take shallower breaths.

Why would this work? "Slow breathing at about this rate exercises the control reflexes that govern our blood pressure and other involuntary functions. They become more efficient and may help prevent an asthma attack," Dr. Lehrer explains.

Breathing Basics

There are dozens of different therapeutic breathing techniques. Here are some simple but powerful exercises to get your breath going.

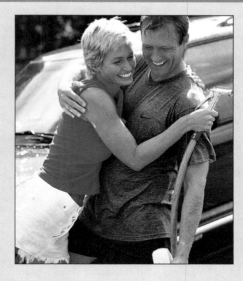

Breathing Coordination

From Carl Stough, founder of the Carl Stough Institute of Breathing Coordination in New York City

Start by doing this exercise lying down. When it becomes easy, try it sitting or standing. Keeping your jaw loose, inhale deeply but comfortably through your mouth. As you exhale, audibly count (a soft whisper is fine). Concentrate on opening your throat muscles as wide as possible so that you can extend the exhalation without any pressure or effort, getting rid of as much carbon dioxide as possible. At the end of the exhalation, you'll inhale automatically because of the vacuum created by your empty lungs. Continue for 10 minutes.

Stough believes that repeatedly practicing this simple exercise is the key to retraining your diaphragm to breathe properly and therefore increasing your oxygen intake. He suggests doing it first thing in the morning and before you go to bed at night, although you may practice it at other times as well.

The Workstation Breathing Break

From Jeffrey A. Migdow, M.D., holistic physician in private practice in Lennox, Massachusetts, and coauthor of Breathe In, Breathe Out: Inhale Energy and Exhale Stress By Guiding and Controlling Your Breathing

Sit up straight with your legs uncrossed. Take slow, deep breaths, allowing your abdomen to fill completely. Exhale as far as possible. Repeat for 1 to 2 minutes. Then, mentally scan your body from head to toe, noting spots that are tense. As you inhale, visualize these areas relaxing as they open and fill with air; as you exhale, feel the aches, pains, and tension being released. Move those tense areas, shrugging your shoulders or wiggling your toes, for example.

Continue the exercise for 2 minutes. For optimal effect, you can repeat this whenever necessary. Because it's fairly subtle, quick, and easy, Dr. Migdow says that it's a perfect stress buster to use at work or in any public place.

cisco State University. Since breathing is one of the few functions in the body that is both voluntary and involuntary, Dr. Peper calls it "a gateway between the conscious and the nonconscious."

"Breath has been used for 5,000 years as the road to consciousness," adds Dr. Goode.

Many cultures associate breath with energy and spirit: The Indian *prana*, the Chinese *chi*, the Japanese *ki*, the Greek *pneuma*, the Latin *spiritus*, and the Hebrew *neshamah* all refer to the air we breathe, or breath itself, as well as to our spirits, souls, and life energy, or essence.

"When you're breathing properly, you're more open to feelings and sensations, and there's a better chance to feel inner connections," explains Dr. Migdow, who lived at a yoga ashram for 15 years. "The only way you can feel a connection to God is to be relaxed enough to get there, and that means optimum breathing."

Breathwork is key to various meditation traditions, not only helping center and calm you but often leading to spiritual insights and even to altered states of consciousness. Breathing meditations are used in Buddhism, Taoism, Tibetan Vajrayana, Sufism, and of course, yoga.

Pranayama yoga is, in fact, the ancient Indian science of breath, designed to optimize the flow of life force throughout the body. Most of the other forms of yoga also depend heavily on manipulating breathing in a variety of ways (speeding it up, slowing it down, holding it) and for a variety of reasons (to relax, rejuvenate, purify, or even heighten sexual response). Zen meditation, on the other hand, seeks only to observe breath, not manipulate it, using it as a focal point to help clear the mind.

Not all spiritual uses of breath come from the East. The ancient Christians used to hold their breath to attain euphoric states during baptism. Jewish Kabbalists visualize God breathing into them as they inhale, just as in the Bible story of God breathing into Adam when he was created. As they exhale, they imagine breathing into God, thus using breath to unite with their Creator.

Chapter 21

Put Massage on Your To-Do List

Enjoy the benefits of do-it-yourself relaxation.

You may think of massage as pure pampering, and that's not a bad thing. But it also offers some physical and psychological bonuses.

"Massage puts you in a relaxed state," says Tiffany Field, Ph.D., director of the Touch Research Institutes at the University of Miami School of Medicine and Nova Southeastern University, which study the effects of massage in five research centers around the world. Not simply a luxurious form of relaxation, massage slows heart rate, lowers blood pressure, reduces stress hormones, and results in overall improved immunity to illness.

The practice of massage is as old as civilization itself. Hieroglyphs demon-

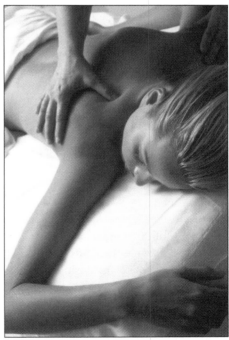

strate that cave dwellers practiced a sort of kneading therapy all over the body. In fact, every corner of the world has some type of traditional massage that precedes the written word. During World War I, massage was used extensively in the treatment of nerve injury and shell shock.

Today, massage is used for everything from relaxation to psychotherapy; its pleasures and benefits are available to everyone.

Massage Basics

Massage is officially defined as the systematic and purposeful manipulation of the soft tissues of the body, which include muscles, connective tissues, even organs—just about everything but bone, says Janet Kahn, Ph.D., a licensed massage therapist and senior research scientist at Wellsley College Center for Research on Women in Takoma Park, Maryland. It can include gentle and stimulating motions: kneading, pressing, rubbing, rolling, tapping, featherlight stroking, and even just touch—the laying on of hands.

There are many different schools or traditions of massage: Swedish, shiatsu (meaning "finger pressure"), and sports massage, just to name some of the more popular types.

"Most massage therapists pick and choose from a variety of forms during a session, depending on their client's needs and preferences," Dr. Kahn says. Massage has proven benefits for people with arthritis, fibromyalgia, chronic fatigue syndrome, back pain, diabetes, cancer, high blood pressure, and carpal tunnel syndrome.

Making Massage Oil Is Fun and Easy

To make a massage oil, combine one of the following carrier oils with one of the essential oils listed below. The mixture ratio is 3 drops of essential oil per ounce of carrier oil. Bottle your creation, label it, and voilà!

Carrier Oils

Sweet almond oil. A pale yellow oil from the kernels of almonds, it contains glucosides, minerals, vitamins, and protein. It may be used on all skin types. When used regularly, it helps to relieve itching, soreness, dryness, and inflammation.

Jojoba oil. A golden oil from the jojoba bean, jojoba oil is great for inflamed skin, psoriasis, eczema, acne, or hair care. Containing protein and minerals, it includes components that mimic collagen. Jojoba is highly penetrative and can be used on all skin types.

Apricot kernel oil. This light yellow oil from the apricot fruit is rich in minerals and vitamins, and is good for all skin types. Prematurely aged, sensitive, inflamed, and dry skin benefit most from this oil.

Olive oil. Deep green and full of protein, minerals, and vitamins, olive oil is good for rheumatic conditions, hair care, and cosmetics. It is soothing to irritated skin.

Grapeseed oil. This green oil is light and delicate, making it a favorite for massage and body applications. It may be used on any type of skin. Grapeseed oil contains vitamins, minerals, and proteins.

Essential Oils

Clary sage. Known as a cell regenerator for aged skin, clary sage is thought to improve the skin's release of natural lubricants. It reputedly stimulates hair growth, soothes inflamed skin, and causes euphoria. Do not use with alcohol; it can cause lethargy and exaggerate drunkenness.

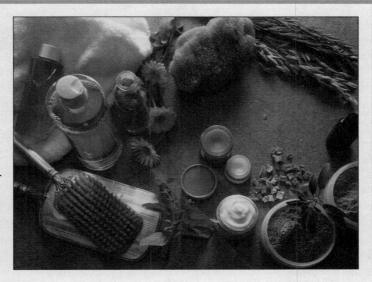

Cypress. This oil stimulates circulation and is great for all kinds of massage. Do not use if you have high blood pressure, cancer, or breast or uterine fibroids.

Eucalyptus. Recognized by aromatherapists as an inhalant to relieve congestion, it can be used topically to reduce sensitivity to muscular pain because of its analgesic properties. Don't use eucalyptus for more than 2 weeks without the guidance of a qualified practitioner, and don't use it at the same time as homeopathic remedies. If you want to try it in the bath, don't add more than three drops to the water. Do not apply to the faces of infants and young children.

Geranium. This oil has a fresh, sweet, slightly floral note and blends well with all citrus oils as well as basil. It's an antiseptic and astringent, so it's thought to be good for acne and aged skin. It's also used for relieving PMS and menopausal tension, and it acts as a stimulant and antidepressant.

Lavender. Used for thousands of years to restore unbalanced states of mind and body, lavender is very calming for insomnia and fluctuating moods. It's also an antiseptic and can help dermatitis, acne, eczema, oily skin, and possibly psoriasis.

Peppermint. Stimulating and uplifting, peppermint is said to be a memory enhancer and to stimulate creativity. Avoid it in the evenings, unless you want to stay awake. It's excellent for foot massage. Do not get it near your eyes. Do not use it on the faces of infants and small children.

How Does It Work?

Our muscles are like stubborn mules that repeat the same old movements every single day, whether good or bad. Massage is introduced to the body to re-educate the muscles.

Manipulating the muscles into new movements, increasing their range of motion, softening the tissue, and lengthening and stretching muscles and connective tissue all change the biomechanical memory of the muscles involved. Overuse or injury to muscle and connective tissue can cause knots or tension clusters. These areas can be slowly released through deep-tissue massage.

Classical Swedish/American neuromuscular massage, which is the most popular type of massage in the United States, affects the interaction between the muscles and the nervous system. Muscles are stimulated through nerve cells to contract and relax. Specialized nerve receptors called proprioceptors receive and transmit information to monitor and protect the soft muscle tissue. Functions like degree of stretch, joint positioning, rate of movement, and muscle tension are all channeled through these receptor sites. Muscle and connective tissue dysfunction is almost always accompanied by proprioceptor hyperactivity that causes the muscle to tense up or become spastic. Opposing muscle groups become involved and, finally, a tight muscle results in a weakened muscle and vice versa.

Besides the basic muscular benefits, massage is an overhaul for the entire body.

> **ONE-MINUTE FAT BURNER**
>
> Call a friend. Fill loneliness with talk—not cookies. Better yet, give each other a massage.

• Circulation is improved. "Massage brings bloodflow to all the body's systems," says Mary Beth Packard, a registered massage therapist practicing in Fort Worth, Texas. "When I'm teaching about massage, I like to start out with talking about bloodflow, because that's the basis for everything." Increased bloodflow encourages more nutrients and oxygen to visit the area being manipulated.

• Improved filtration and elimination of carbon dioxide encourages your organs and cells to do their work more efficiently. Don't be surprised if you notice that your digestion and skin tone improve after a massage, says Packard.

• Massage can also act as a mechanical cleaner, hastening the elimination of waste and toxic debris, such as lactic acid and uric acid, that are stored in your muscles, especially after exercise, Dr. Kahn says. "If you get a massage soon after your workout, your muscles get less achy and stiff," she adds.

• A massage is a good way to feel more positive about your body image. "Very often, I have women tell me that they were apprehensive about coming in for a massage because they are overweight. But after one session, they're completely comfortable with it," says Packard. "Massage is a great body-awareness tool, a good way to get back in touch with your body."

• Massage soothes the nervous system and is an integral part of stress management. "As the body relaxes, it goes from a sympathetic to a more sleepful parasympathetic state," says Susan Norris, a certified massage therapist and holistic practitioner at the Beauty Kliniek in San Diego. "This takes the body from fight-or-flight mode to a more relaxed state. Neurotransmitters release endorphins as a result of the manipulation of muscle tissue. The endorphins released allow for a feeling of well-being."

• Studies confirm that massage can improve the quality of your sleep. "A back rub before bedtime used to be standard care for hospital patients, and it really did help people to relax and sleep better," says Arline Reinking-Hanf, R.N., a massage therapist for the Complementary Care Service Center at the New York–Presbyterian Hospital in New York.

To benefit the most from a massage, Adina Moldovan, a certified massage therapist at Tova's in Houston, advises, "Don't drink alcohol or caffeinated beverages for 24 hours before getting a massage, and drink plenty of water after the massage to cleanse the system of toxins released from the deep tissues and muscles." To make the benefits of massage last, you must continue to support the balance in the body that has been created by the massage, she says. Deep breathing, a natural diet, plenty of sleep, and keeping the body clear of toxins like nicotine and food preservatives are all required to extend the positive effects of massage.

How Is It Done?

Initially, your massage therapist should ask you some questions, including whether this is your first massage, what your reasons are for wanting a massage, and if you have any health problems.

Then you'll be asked to take off whatever

A Word of Caution

Even though massage is of enormous benefit, never receive a massage when you have the following conditions unless given your doctor's permission.

- An infection, high body temperature, or a contagious or systemic disease
- Acute back pain, especially if the pain shoots down your arms or legs when you receive touch to your back
- A skin infection, bruising, or acute inflammation
- An inflammatory condition such as thrombosis or phlebitis

---

clothes you feel comfortable removing and to climb under a sheet or large towel draped over a comfortable, padded massage table. If you're getting shiatsu, you might not remove any clothes, and you may be asked to lie on a mat on the floor. Proper massage etiquette requires that only the part of your body being massaged be exposed. Most therapists use oil or lotion. They may start anywhere on your body, but they are more likely to start on your back, head, or feet. They may work over your whole body or may concentrate on certain parts, depending on what you want. "It's important to communicate with your massage therapist about what you want and what feels good or bad," Dr. Kahn says.

A typical session may last 45 minutes to an hour. People who are very frail or sick, however,

(continued on page 196)

Self-Massage for What Ails You

Practitioners agree that for optimum benefit—to relieve stress and ease stiff, sore muscles—nothing beats regular, professional massage. But with a little practice, you can give yourself an effective massage and treat yourself when time and money are short, according to Susan Edwards, a licensed massage therapist, co-owner of and instructor at the Somerset School of Massage in New Jersey, and author of *The Healing Power of Self-Massage*.

"When you need to relax right now, self-massage is as close as your fingertips," says Edwards.

Here is a step-by-step guide to get you started with a simple self-massage.

Place the inner sides of your thumbs against the bony sockets surrounding your eyes, starting with the tip of your thumbs next to the bridge of your nose. Put your forefingers on top of the edges of the sockets, just below your eyebrows. Lightly press against the bone with your thumbs, holding for 5 to 10 seconds. Release the pressure and move your fingers a bit, slowly working your way to the outside corners of the sockets. Be sure to release the pressure from your fingers before moving them so that you don't drag your fingers along the delicate skin surrounding your eyes.

Place all of your fingers together in two side-by-side vertical lines on the middle of your forehead, letting your thumbs rest on your temples. Press lightly with your fingers for 5 to 10 seconds and release. Move your fingers about 1 inch apart and repeat. Continue until you cover your entire forehead. Be careful not to press too hard.

Place your middle fingers on your temples and your thumbs on your jawbone for support. Gently massage your temples on both sides of your head by rotating your middle fingers upward and backward, away from your eyes, for 15 seconds. You can also use the same movement to massage your jaws and around your ears.

Press with your right thumb into the lower part of the palm of your left hand in line with your left little finger, making small rotations with firm pressure. Then, going clockwise, use your thumb to massage around your palm in a circle. When you reach the top of your palm, concentrate on the fleshy spaces in between the bones. Repeat on the other hand.

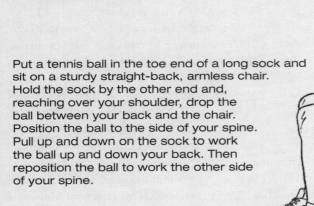

Put a tennis ball in the toe end of a long sock and sit on a sturdy straight-back, armless chair. Hold the sock by the other end and, reaching over your shoulder, drop the ball between your back and the chair. Position the ball to the side of your spine. Pull up and down on the sock to work the ball up and down your back. Then reposition the ball to work the other side of your spine.

Sitting on a sturdy armless chair, rest your ankle on your opposite thigh, and with lengthwise or circular motions, use your thumbs to work all over the sole of your foot. Then massage across the top of your foot with your thumbs, working from your ankle down to your toes and up the side of your foot from your big toe to your inner ankle. Repeat on your other foot.

may do better with shorter, more frequent sessions of 20 to 30 minutes, Dr. Kahn says.

Most forms of massage are extremely pleasant and relaxing. Sometimes, a massage therapist will apply pressure over a knotted muscle and produce what is called good pain, which quickly fades as the muscle relaxes. During your massage, you should feel calm and nurtured. Afterward, you should feel calm and energized.

One massage session may reduce your pain for a few hours or days, and regular massage sessions may help keep certain types of pain at bay for long periods of time and even improve your muscle performance, Dr. Kahn says. One study conducted by researchers at the Group Health Center for Health Studies and the University of Washington, both in Seattle, and the Center for Alternative Medicine Research in Boston found that people with lower-back pain who got up to 10 massages had less pain and improved ability to function compared with people who got acupuncture or just educational materials after 10 weeks of treatment.

Who's Qualified to Do It?

Roughly 29 states and the District of Columbia regulate massage therapists, and all of those states have a minimum training requirement. To find out if your state has licensing requirements, call your state regulatory office or contact the American Massage Therapy Association (AMTA) at 820 Davis Street, Suite 100, Evanston, IL 60201-4400. This organization can also provide the names of AMTA members near you.

Massage therapists can also be nationally certified. As a member of AMTA, a massage therapist has a minimum of 500 hours training from a school accredited by the Commission on Massage Therapy Accreditation or a member of the AMTA Council of Schools, plus continuing education, and carries malpractice liability insurance. For a professional massage, prices range from $45 to $100-plus for a 60-minute session. Prices are higher in urban areas and on the East and West coasts, and lower in the rural Midwest.

Chapter 22

How to Get the Rest You Crave

The right amount of sleep can improve how you think, look, and feel—overnight.

It's every woman's most powerful bedroom fantasy: a good night's sleep.

The average woman sleeps 6 hours and 41 minutes a night during the workweek, according to the National Sleep Foundation's 1998 Women and Sleep Poll (WSP). Meanwhile, research indicates that almost everyone needs 8 hours and 12 minutes a night.

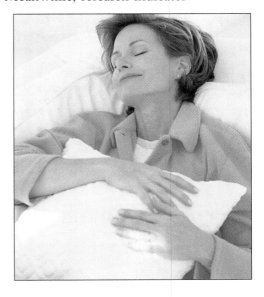

Is it any wonder that 3 out of 10 women in the poll said their sleep deficit frequently interferes with daily activities? Sleep deprivation cuts energy levels, reduces your ability to concentrate, and can make you moody, affecting everything from your work performance to your relationships to your driving skills. The overnight remedy for most of us is 8 solid hours of rest.

While You Were Sleeping

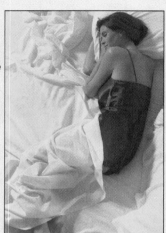

Sleep is a process, not a single, static state. As you drift off, you enter stage one, very light sleep. Your muscles start to relax, but your brain waves are still rapid and unpredictable. If the phone were to ring, you would sit right up.

At stage two, brain waves become larger as you sink into a more profound slumber. By stages three and four, your brain produces slow, big, even waves; your heart rate and respiration slow; and your blood pressure lowers. In this deep stage of sleep, your body works to heal and restore itself.

After about an hour in stage four, you begin a fifth stage, characterized by rapid eye movement (REM). Your brain gets very active; the waves are almost identical to those you experience when awake. Now you dream.

You cycle in and out of REM sleep several times during the night, and each successive REM period is longer than the last. During these times, you're essentially paralyzed, which prevents you from hurting yourself or your bedmate during action-packed nocturnal head trips.

REM sleep is also when your brain does its filing—sorting, storing, and discarding the day's memories. That's why sleep deprivation quickly causes problems in mood and memory: You need nighttime processing for your brain to function efficiently the next day.

Even if you're certain you can't squeeze more sleep hours out of your day, here's how you can learn to sleep more efficiently.

‖ The Sleepless Sex

Most of us cling to the mistaken notion that we can make do with less shut-eye. But scientists have found that nothing can change a person's fundamental daily snooze requirement. Some of us naturally need 9 hours, while a lucky few can get away with 6 to 7 hours.

Women in general seem to need more rest than men. "In studies in which people are allowed to wake up whenever they want, we find that women rise from 20 to 50 minutes later than men," says Helen Driver, Ph.D., a sleep researcher at Toronto Western Hospital.

Yet in real life, women are the more sleepless sex, getting an average of 34 minutes less shut-eye than men. Why? Women's hormonal changes seem to negatively affect sleep, as do our towering stress loads, says Amy Wolfson, Ph.D., associate professor of psychology at College of the Holy Cross in Worcester, Massachusetts. "The majority of women work full-time, but most are still responsible for the care of the home. They neglect sleep as a result."

Exhaustion, always inconvenient, can turn catastrophic. Every year, the day after we turn our clocks ahead for daylight savings time, auto accidents increase by 7 percent. The Challenger explosion, the Chernobyl meltdown, and the Exxon Valdez oil spill have all been linked to human error that resulted from sleep deprivation. Without enough rest, cognitive ability suffers, memory dims, and susceptibility to infection increases.

‖ Snooze Snatchers

A variety of factors, both physical and psychological, can eat up your sleep time, says Martin Moore-Ede, M.D., Ph.D., chief executive officer of Circadean Technologies, a Cambridge, Massachusetts, research and consulting firm specializing in reducing workplace fatigue, and coauthor of *The Complete Idiot's Guide to Getting a Good Night's Sleep*.

Common lifestyle-related causes of sleep problems include drinking alcohol or caffeinated drinks late in the evening, eating foods before going to bed that could cause heartburn, arguing with your mate before bedtime, worrying about

Weight Loss
HELP OR HYPE?

Hypnotize Pounds Off?

Are you wondering if hypnosis can help you lose weight? Don't count on it.

A better choice would be a cognitive/behavioral therapist who will teach you how to make diet, exercise, and lifestyle changes that will help you lose weight.

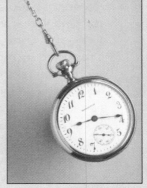

David B. Allison, Ph.D., of the Obesity Research Center at St. Luke's–Roosevelt Hospital Center in New York City, found that to be true when he evaluated studies comparing the effectiveness of hypnosis combined with cognitive/behavioral therapy to the therapy alone. People who received hypnosis did not lose more weight than those not undergoing hypnosis, he says.

To find what will work best for you, ask yourself why you're interested in hypnosis. If you're looking for support, join a weight-loss group such as TOPS (Take Off Pounds Sensibly). Looking for a quick fix? Sorry, there really is none.

Diagnose It: What's Keeping You Up?

These questions should help you pin-point your specific sleep issues.

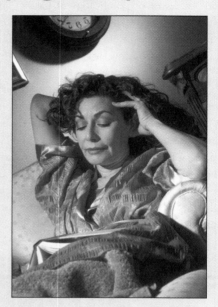

1. Do you have a hard time falling asleep but slumber well once you've drifted off? Stress is the most likely culprit. In the National Sleep Foundation's Women and Sleep Poll (WSP), 34 percent of women said that stress affected their sleep. Caffeine or nicotine close to bedtime may also be contributing to the problem.

2. Do you repeatedly wake up at night? Avoid alcohol close to bedtime. Liquor-induced sleep is not as restful as natural sleep, and when the alcohol wears off, you're likely to awaken suddenly. Also see #3.

3. Do you snore or gasp during the night? You may have sleep apnea, in which the tissue in your throat and upper airway collapses while you are in deep sleep. Then your brain suddenly screams, "Wake up!" and you start breathing again. Since this happens repeatedly during the night, sleep is fragmented and much less restful. Apnea is reported by more men than women, though after age 50, both genders suffer from it equally. Remedies include sleeping on your side, losing weight (if you are heavy), and avoiding nighttime use of alcohol, tobacco, and sleeping pills. Surgery to increase the size of the airway is also an option.

4. Are you always tired, even when you get a solid 8 hours? Going to bed and getting up at different times every day (yes, even on lazy weekends) can take a toll on your sleep quality. Constant exhaustion can be a symptom of depression, too.

5. Are you menopausal or perimenopausal? Women going through menopause tie with pregnant women for the greatest number of sleep problems. In the WSP, 36 percent of menopausal women reported hot flashes that disrupted sleep. Discuss the pros and cons of estrogen-replacement therapy with your doctor.

unfinished business from the workday, and engaging in vigorous exercise after 6:00 or 7:00 P.M. (Experts say that having sex is the exception to this rule.) A bedroom that is too light or either too hot or cold, and an uncomfortable bed are also likely to stand between you and dreamtime.

The quality of your sleep is a barometer of your health. Insomnia can result from depression, pain, or sleep apnea, a condition that causes you to stop breathing for anywhere from 10 to 60 seconds at a time, then wake up for a few moments, then fall back asleep—sometimes without even being aware that your sleep has been disturbed. Restless Leg Syndrome, which makes your legs feel so jumpy that you have to move them to get relief, can also keep you awake. Here are some other culprits you might never have suspected.

Your meds. Insomnia can be caused by some common drugs, including those for colds and allergies (like Sudafed, Actifed, and Robitussin CF). Medication for high blood pressure, heart disease, and asthma can compromise sleep, too, as can progesterone-based birth control medications, like medroxyprogesterone (Depo-Provera). Read the label of your over-the-counter (OTC) pain reliever; a few, such as Excedrin, contain caffeine.

Your partner. If he snores, that is. A Mayo Clinic study showed that when men with sleep apnea were fitted with devices to stop their snoring, their partners got more than an hour of extra sleep per night, on average.

Your period. Half of all menstruating women experience sleep problems. Poor sleep quality is most likely to occur at the beginning of your cycle (day 1 being the day bleeding starts) for a variety of reasons, including simple cramps. In addition, the hormone progesterone, which rises after ovulation (around day 14), may cause some women to feel more fatigued. Around day 21, progesterone levels start to drop, which may make it hard to fall asleep. Around days 22 to 28, if you're susceptible to premenstrual syndrome, you may experience a variety of symptoms ranging from insomnia to hypersomnia (sleeping too much) to daytime tiredness. Research suggests that women who have PMS spend only 5 percent of their total sleep time in the deeply restorative stage-three and stage-four sleep, while those without PMS spend 15 to 20 percent in megaslumber.

Your commute. Suburbanites have it rough, according to a study of commuters on the Long Island Rail Road by Joyce Walseben, Ph.D., director of the Sleep Disorders Center at New York University. Study participants who commuted more than an hour and 15 minutes each way averaged 30 minutes less sleep a night than those with shorter commutes. More than 50 percent reported having problems sleeping once in bed or staying awake during the day. Dr. Walseben says commuter trains should feature dimmed lights and a no-talking policy.

Your hours. Those who work nontraditional hours (20 percent of all Americans) have more trouble falling asleep than those who work standard shifts, according to Jodi Mindell, Ph.D., a sleep researcher and professor of psychology at St. Joseph's University in Philadelphia and author of *Sleeping Through the Night*. "Our circadian rhythms and biological clocks are governed by

1-MINUTE FAT BURNER

Reflect on your choices. Looking at yourself in a mirror while eating may help you consume 22 to 32 percent less food.

light, and shift workers are often working when their bodies want to be sleeping."

Turning Out the Lights, Naturally

Rest easy. There are lots of things you can do to ensure a blissful night's sleep. Here are some snooze supporters from the experts.

Make time. Allow yourself at least 45 minutes to an hour to unwind before you lie down in bed. Avoid working on finances, watching the late news, or stimulating your mind in any way too close to bedtime.

Don't be a clock watcher. Remove your clock from your bedside. In fact, remove it from the room, if possible. If it's your alarm clock, cover up the face.

Cozy up. Create a comfortable bed and

Rx for Great Sleep

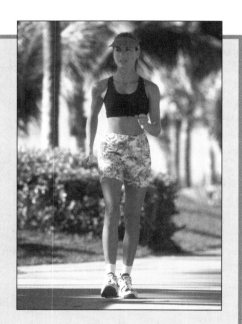

A mere six-block stroll can take you a long way toward sounder slumber. When more than 700 men and women were asked about their exercise and sleep habits, the researchers discovered that walkers had fewer sleep-related problems such as waking in the middle of the night, nightmares, and feeling tired around 3:00 P.M.

Compared to those who didn't walk at all, people who walked at least six blocks a day at a normal pace were one-third less likely to have trouble sleeping until their wake-up time. Those who walked the same distance at a brisk pace slashed the risk of any sleep disorder by 50 percent.

Walking is such an effective sleep aid that "we frequently tell people with insomnia to walk for a half-hour during the day," says study coauthor Stuart Quan, M.D., of the Respiratory Sciences and Sleep Disorders Center at the University of Arizona College of Medicine in Tucson.

For many people, walking works just as well as medication, and without side effects such as morning grogginess, risk of sleep apnea, and possible addiction. It also helps you avoid the common sleep disturbances that occur as you get older. It's best to avoid heart-pounding workouts for at least 2 hours before bed, however. Vigorous exercise may make it harder to fall asleep.

Herbal Sleepytime Pillow

Using miniature handmade pillows stuffed with sleep-inducing herbs is a time-honored path to dreamland. And these pillows work well for everyone, including children and the elderly, says Phoebe Reeve, a professional member of the American Herbalists Guild and an herbalist in Winchester, Virginia. "It's something that's beautiful and natural, and that in itself is soothing," she says. "Plus, the scent is physiologically and psychologically soporific." That means that the fragrance is relaxing for body and soul.

If you can't find all of these dried herbs, any combination or even just one can help you sleep better. The pillow is not meant to cradle your whole head when you sleep; instead, just place it near your nose when you lie down. "It's also something nice to hold on to while you sleep," says Reeve.

1 tablespoon lavender (*Lavandula spp.*)

1 tablespoon chamomile (*Matricaria recutita*)

1 tablespoon hops (*Humulus lupulus*)

1 tablespoon mugwort (*Artemisia vulgaris*)

1 tablespoon rose (*Rosa spp.*)

Cut two small rectangles of the same size from a cotton fabric, such as muslin (Reeve recommends 4 inches × 4 inches, but you can make yours a bit bigger if you prefer). Making sure that the right sides are facing each other, sew the fabric together on three sides. Turn the pieces inside-out.

Using the lavender, chamomile, hops, mugwort, and rose singly or in any combination, stuff the pillow, then sew it closed.

To reactivate the scent of the herbs, sprinkle vodka or any odorless grain alcohol on the pillow and let it dry. Your pillow should remain effective for about a year; you can then refill it with a new batch of herbs.

bedroom. From room temperature to the crispness of the sheets to the fluffiness of your pillow, everything should be just the way you like it when you turn in for the night.

Sip a natural relaxer. Tranquilizing herbal tea blends made with chamomile, valerian, or passionflower are age-old sleep aids for their ability to induce drowsiness, while warm milk contains tryptophan, a chemical that also helps make you sleepy, says Dr. Moore-Ede.

Play up pleasure. Off with the car chases, bad sitcoms, and general blare of the TV, and on with soft music, a traditional relaxation tool. Choose jazz, classical, R&B—whatever style you prefer, as long as it's smooth and mellow. Tuning in should help you tune out your troubles. Prayer and meditation can also bring peace and allow you to shut off the cares of the day.

Drift off. Reading poetry, short stories, or other relaxing fare can help get you ready for dreamland. Those who have a really hard time

How Much Sleep Do You Really Need?

The Sleep Foundation has a Web site (www.sleepfoundation.org/publications/diary.html) with a diary that you can print out and use to track your exercise, eating, and drinking habits; your bedtime activities; and your retiring and waking times. Once you've recorded your patterns and levels of tiredness for a few weeks, you'll get a sense of which routines interfere with your sleep.

falling asleep should probably avoid thrillers and scary science fiction.

Immerse yourself. Slipping into a warm bath for 20 minutes can ease the transition from a stressful day to a quiet evening. As the heat relaxes tired muscles, let your mind drift to pleasant thoughts, says Meir Kryger, M.D., past president of the American Sleep Disorders Foundation and professor of medicine at the University of Manitoba-Winnipeg.

Get into a rhythm. Practicing rhythmic breathing can help take your focus off your mind and direct it toward your body. Simply breathe deeply, filling first your stomach and then your lungs with air; and exhale slowly, allowing yourself to become more drowsy and calm each time you exhale.

Stretch your limits. Stretching or tensing your muscles one at a time for a few seconds and then relaxing them helps release tension. And a relaxed body is one that will drift off to sleep easily, says Dr. Kryger.

‖ When All Else Fails

What if, despite all your best efforts, you still can't fall asleep? Should you take medication? "Sleeping pills and tranquilizers can be helpful in the short-term," says Peter Hauri, Ph.D., codirector of the Sleep Disorders Center at the Mayo Clinic.

"They allow you to get to sleep if you're in a different time zone and absolutely need to be well-rested and alert, or if there's been a death in the family and the grief and stress have made it impossible for you to sleep. But if you're taking them more than once or twice a week, that may be a problem," cautions Dr. Hauri. When your inability to sleep interferes seriously with your daytime functioning for more than a month or two, it's time to seek professional help, he notes.

Indeed, if your insomnia is chronic, you should try to work your way around medication. "You're far better off dealing with the environmental and lifestyle issues that are likely to be keeping you awake," says Dr. Moore-Ede.

Catnap

There's evidence that even a 15- to 20-minute daytime nap can increase alertness, revive memory, and reduce the symptoms of fatigue. Limit your sleep to less than an hour, however, or you'll wake up groggy and compromise your nighttime sleep. Schedule your snooze for sometime between 2:00 and 4:00 P.M., when your circadian rhythms are most conducive to slumber.

LIFESTYLE RESTYLE

She Used Her Mind to Slim Her Body

After years of dieting, Leigh Anne Congdon finally took off—and kept off—30 pounds. She did it, she says, by learning how to think like a thin person.

As a teenager, Congdon was unhappy with her body. She was only a few pounds overweight, but she saw herself as chunky and unattractive. She'd go on self-styled diets of less than 1,000 calories a day for a couple of weeks, each time losing a few pounds. But once she returned to her normal eating habits, the weight always came back.

This cycle of gaining, losing, and regaining continued through high school and college. Then, Congdon made a decision that would turn her eating habits upside down. "When I graduated from college, I moved from Pennsylvania to Colorado with a group of friends," she explains. "I thought that I could find a job out there, and I was excited about living in another part of the country. I needed the change."

Away from home and living with her friends, Congdon decided it was time to enjoy herself. That meant not worrying about what she was eating. She joined her friends in a steady diet of pizza, burgers, barbecued ribs, and other "forbidden" foods that she had deprived herself of for so long. Within a year, her weight climbed from 140 to 160 pounds—too heavy for her 5-foot-5-inch frame.

Once again, Congdon decided that it was time for a fresh start. "It wasn't only my weight," she says. "It was the part-time jobs, the small apartments. I needed some direction in my life."

She headed back East, enrolled in graduate school, and committed to slimming down healthfully and permanently.

Remembering how dieting had failed her in the past, but not wanting to monitor every bite of food that she put in her mouth, Congdon decided to change her mindset. "I had noticed that my friends who were thin didn't constantly dwell on what they were eating," she explains. "They ate when they were hungry and said, 'No, thanks' when they weren't. I followed their example and tried to stop obsessing about food. I resolved to think like a thin person. I'd eat a little bit of something and then tell myself that I was full, because that's what a thin person would do."

She ate healthier, too, and increased her activity level, believing that a thin person would be active.

With her new "thin" attitude, Congdon was able to take off 30 pounds in about 9 months. Now age 42, she has maintained her weight at a healthy 130 pounds ever since.

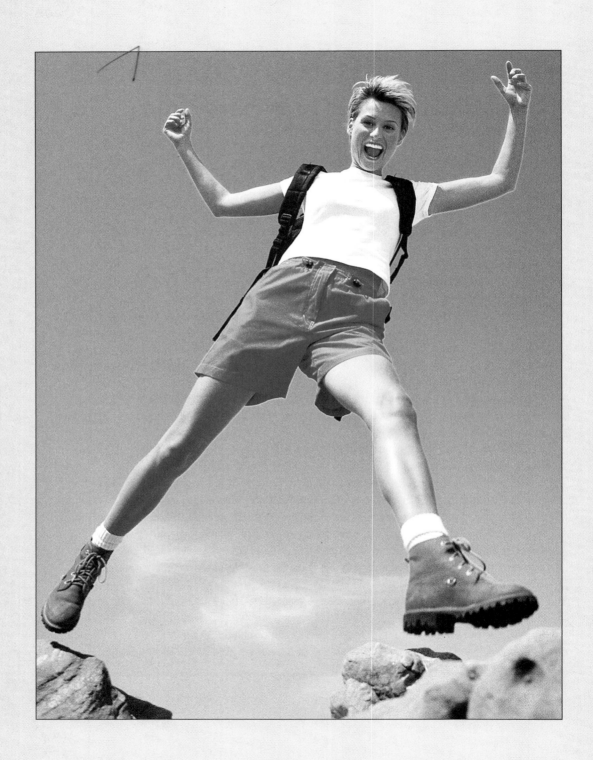

Part Six

Age Erasers
for Real Women

Chapter 23

Look 10 Pounds Slimmer—Today

You can find clothes that flatter your figure *now.*

Imagine getting dressed in the late 19th century. You wrap whalebone around your waist, suck in your stomach, and hang on to the bedposts while someone tightens your corset. If you're a tight lacer, you don't quit until your waist measures a fashionable 14 inches.

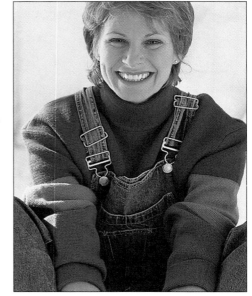

Luckily, you don't need bones and strings to look thinner in today's world. Nor do you have to wait until you actually lose as much weight as you want to enjoy the benefits of looking thinner.

A certain color, a particular cut, or a specific fabric is all it takes to minimize your hips and thighs, shrink your waist, and give you more height. It's simply a matter of knowing how to create the illusion.

Start with Your Mirror

Stand at least a body length away from a full-length mirror in a well-lit area—totally naked. "It's like being in a museum," says Laurie Krauz, an image consultant in New York City. "You get to see the entire artwork."

Are you tall or short? Broad or narrow? Is the line from your shoulder to your hip straight, or is it curvy? "Instead of trying to fix your body," Krauz explains, "you need to learn your body. Understand the line of your body so you can select clothing that agrees with that line."

To do that, you need to determine your body shape. There are four body shapes: pear, hourglass, apple, and rectangle. To narrow your choices, look at your waist.

"I call them waist or waist-nots," says Catherine Schuller, a New York City–based fashion retail editor of *Mode* magazine and author of *The Ultimate Plus-Size Modeling Guide*. "Either you have an indentation above your hips or you're straight up and down." If you have an indentation, you're a pear or an hourglass. If you don't, you're an apple or a rectangle.

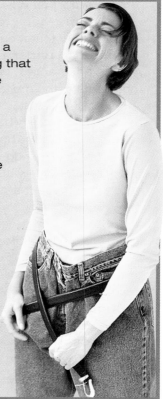

Get Rid of Your "Fat Dress"

It might be a pair of jeans, a roomy sweatshirt, or even a dress—your "fat dress." We all have one. It's something that we wore at our biggest. You probably hang yours in the back of your closet and feel comforted that it's there in case of emergency.

"I have clients who have three different types of clothes in their closet: current clothes, thin clothes, and fat clothes," says Jan Larkey, a Pittsburgh-based image consultant and author of *Flatter Your Figure*.

But you've made a commitment to lose weight now. Here are a few creative and liberating ways to put your fat clothes to rest.

• Cut them up, turn them into a collage, and frame it as a constant reminder of why you're changing your lifestyle.

• Make them into a quilt or a throw pillow.

• Cut them up into rags, then burn calories by cleaning your house or waxing your car with them.

• Donate them to an organization that provides career clothes to poor women.

Flatten Your Belly by Tonight

Do you need to look your slimmest—fast? These debloating and camouflaging tricks can take an inch or more off your waistline in 12 hours.

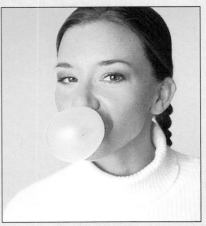

Drink water. Carbonated drinks and those with lots of sugar can blow your belly up like a balloon, says Peter McNally, D.O., spokesperson for the American College of Gastroenterology.

Skip the chips. Salt makes you retain water, especially before your period. Processed and canned foods tend to be high in sodium.

Give your jaw a break. Chewing gum can cause you to swallow excess air.

Get some java "to go." If you're feeling overdue for a bathroom session, studies show that a cup or two of coffee can get things moving.

Shape up underneath. Body shapers, or high-waisted spandex waist nippers and panties, can take off an inch or more. The more spandex (Lycra) they contain, the more control you'll get.

Note: Excess bulge can squeeze up and over, so avoid clingy tops, says Jan Larkey, a Pittsburgh-based image consultant and author of *Flatter Your Figure*.

Buy the dress that fits now. Forget sizes. No one will see the tag, but if your outfit is too snug around your middle, you might as well yell, "Hey, check out my belly!" Show off your strongest feature to draw attention away from your tummy. Great arms? Go sleeveless. Tina Turner legs? Wear a shorter hemline. Sexy shoulders? Choose thin—or no—straps. If you prefer a dressy suit, choose a long jacket worn over a straight, slim skirt.

Wear "your" color. Don't worry about what's "in"; wear the shade that looks good on you. And keep your outfit monochromatic—same color top, skirt or trousers, and shoes—for an elongating effect, says Princess Jenkins, an image consultant at Majestic Images in New York City.

Choose belly-slimming fabrics. Silks, rayons, knits, and nonclingy matte jerseys generally provide the best results.

Accessorize. Choose eye-catching earrings and necklaces or colorful scarves. They'll draw attention to your face.

Step out in heels. Wearing high heels can make you look taller and thinner.

Here's a full description of each body shape.

The Pear: You have an indentation above your hips. Your waist is 10 to 12 inches smaller than your hips. Most of your weight is distributed below your waist.

The Hourglass: You have an indentation above your hips. Your weight is evenly distributed between your bust and hips.

The Apple: You do not have an indentation above your hips. Your waistline is the widest part of your body. You have thin arms and legs.

The Rectangle: You do not have an indentation above your hips. Your hips, bust, and waist are in proportion to each other.

Once you've figured out your shape, accept it, says Jan Larkey, a Pittsburgh-based image consultant and author of *Flatter Your Figure*. No matter how much weight you gain and lose, your basic structure won't change.

Shop 'til You Drop

Now comes the fun part: choose new clothes that most flatter *your* body type.

Frame your face. "One of the kindest things we can do for ourselves is to wear a collar," says Judith Rasband, an image consultant in Orem, Utah, and author of *Fabulous Fit* and *Wardrobe Strategies for Women*. It lifts people's attention to our faces and away from our bodies.

Choose a V-neck collar because the vertical line is very slimming to everyone, says Claudia Kaneb, wardrobe head at NBC's *Today* show in New York City. For the same effect, wear a long chain with a small pendant or a knotted scarf draped down like a necklace over a shirt with a high collar.

Waist not, want not. Your body type will determine the clothes you choose to minimize your waistline. Follow these guidelines.

Pear: Keep patterns and textures above your waistline and solid colors beneath. "Anything loud or bulky below the waist adds dimension," Schuller says. Wear skirts and pants without pleats.

Hourglass: You're evenly proportioned, says Schuller. You can wear the same clothes as a pear-shaped woman, and you can wear patterns below your waistline.

If you have a flat stomach, try a fluted trumpet skirt. Its long, straight style, flaring out from midcalf to ankle, is very slimming, says Princess Jenkins, an image consultant at Majestic Images International in New York City.

Apple: Look for clothes with an overall downward taper stopping at the end of the garment, whether it's at the bottom hem of a blouse, skirt, or even a sleeve, says Schuller. You are as wide as your widest line, wherever that falls. Avoid horizontal stripes since they add dimension and make you look wider.

Rectangle: Schuller suggests that you choose column dresses that go straight up and down and don't taper. Try fabrics such as velveteen, matte jerseys, and heavy silks, all of which move as your body moves, creating fluidity.

Get hip. At the hips, avoid horizontal lines such as sideways stripes, Jenkins says, because they add weight to every shape. Clothes that slim your hips include A-line skirts, long jackets that cover the hips, loose-fitting tunic tops, and slightly padded shoulders.

To minimize your thighs, Jenkins suggests choosing pants with a semi-full leg, staying away from those that taper at the bottom.

Scale the fashion heights. If you're short, don't wear long shirts over long skirts, Larkey says. Your waist will get lost and you will look even shorter. Accentuate your waist instead with an A-line blazer or belt, and wear skirts that show an extra inch or two above your ankles.

Or try pantsuits, says Kaneb. For those over 5 foot 4, pantsuits with longer jackets that cover hips and thighs make all body types look taller and slimmer.

Find the right fabrics. Anyone carrying extra weight should avoid fabrics such as fleece, tweeds, leather, metallics, and nubby knits, which add visual pounds, Jenkins says. Also stay away from "busy" patterns like large floral prints, checks, and polka dots.

‖ Make It Fit

The right fit helps those fabulous clothes hang well on your body and do what they were meant to do: create an illusion of thinness. "If you wear things too tight, you look large," says Schuller. "If you wear things too big, you look large."

It won't be easy. Designers cut clothes for the proportional woman, someone who is eight heads tall (her head is exactly one-eighth of the length of her body), with shoulders and hips of the same width. So finding clothes that fit *your* body, not Cindy Crawford's, can be a real challenge, especially since the same size may be cut differently by different manufacturers.

But don't give up. "Women go shopping, put something on, it doesn't fit, and they blame

> ## 1-MINUTE FAT BURNER
>
> **Ditch diet shakes. The calorie savings are only temporary; you just eat more later.**

their bodies," Krauz says. "Instead, women should realize that it's the fault of the manufacturer."

Here are some ways to get the right fit every time.

Give yourself enough room. No matter what your figure type, don't wear clothes that cling. A loose fit won't outline the bulges our figures acquire as we age, Rasband says.

Shop for separates. "It's ridiculous to design clothing for women where the top and the bottom are the same size," Krauz says. "The only women it works for are the symmetrical body types."

Search different departments. Don't be afraid to go between the Junior, Misses', and Women's departments for the clothes you need. For instance, blouses in the larger, Women's sizes tend to have bigger armholes. So if you're an apple, you may need to buy your tops in the Women's department and your skirts in the Misses' department, says Larkey. If you're a pear, you may do just the opposite.

Give it the fit test. Once you've found clothes that seem to fit well, put them to the test, says Jenkins. Roll your shoulders forward and make sure the fabric doesn't pull. Raise your arms and make sure you have a comfortable reach. Check that the buttons and zippers are not pulling at the chest or hips.

Get it tailored. You might have to take measures beyond the department store for a good fit. While men can get a suit altered anywhere, women usually have to search for a seamstress and pay extra.

But it's a worthwhile expense, Jenkins says,

because fit is so important. Once you own a piece of clothing that fits perfectly, she says, you'll never want to wear another ill-fitting garment again.

It's All in the Details

Details are why we love to shop. Color, style, and that special something are what makes an outfit truly ours. Those same details can help camouflage many imperfections.

Choose the right color. Color makes a statement. Color has energy. And color can be slimming. "Everybody thinks black is the only color that's slimming," says Mari Lyn Henry, professional member of the Association of Image Consultants International in Washington, D.C. "That's nonsense. If you wear a solid color—dark green, wine red, navy blue, royal purple, teal—it molds to your body and gives you a shadow effect." Vibrant colors can add youthfulness, while light, washed-out colors tend to age you.

Be color consistent. To look thinner, wear a top and bottom of the same or similar color, Jenkins suggests. Splitting your body in half with dark pants and a light-colored shirt makes you look wider.

Up Where They Belong

Hands down, the biggest mistake women make is buying bras that don't fit, says Berna Goldstein, vice president of merchandising for Bali Company bra manufacturer in New York City. "Bras come in many, many different cuts and styles. Just as you can't wear every size-12 pants you put on,

you can't expect that every 36C bra will fit you the way it should." Here's how to get the best wear out of your underwear.

Measure up. A surprising number of women have never had their bra size measured, Goldstein says. "They just buy what they've always bought, which may or may not be the right size and style."

The best plan: Go to an undergarment specialty store and have a salesperson size you properly. But you can also measure yourself. First, find your bra size by measuring around your rib cage directly beneath your bust and adding 5 to the measurement. Next, measure the circumference around your full bust. The difference between the rib-cage and full-bust measurements indicates your bust size.

If you wear a solid color, it molds to your body and gives you a shadow effect.

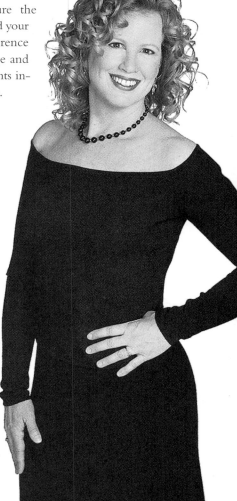

Bolster Your Bustline to Look Younger and Feel Thinner—Instantly

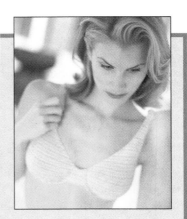

Want to take off 10 pounds and 10 years? It's easier than you think. All you need is the right bra.

"When a bra doesn't fit properly, it either allows breasts to sag too low or it bunches them in so they bulge out of the top and the sides. Both problems can add about 10 pounds and 10 years to a woman's appearance," says Berna Goldstein, vice president of merchandising for Bali Company bra manufacturer in New York City. "And the problem is common. When we survey women, we find that 70 to 85 percent of women are wearing the wrong size or the wrong style bras for their figures."

Ill-fitting bras are especially common among larger-sized women—the ones who can benefit most from the slimming effects of the right bustline support, says Goldstein. "You see many full-figured women who wear bras that let their breasts fall down to their waists. It makes them look much older, heavier, and short-waisted than if they were wearing properly fitted bras that put their breasts up where they belong."

Plus, a bra that provides proper support—especially when you're exercising—can help prevent the supportive ligaments from stretching and causing your breasts to sag in the first place.

Difference	Cup Size
½ inch	AA
1 inch	A
2 inches	B
3 inches	C
4 inches	D
5 inches	DD or E
6 inches	DDD or F
7 inches	FF or G

Fill up without overfilling. When you put on a bra, each cup should completely contain each breast. "If the cup wrinkles or sags anywhere, it's too big," says Goldstein. If you bulge over the top or the sides, you have the wrong size or the wrong style. "If the bra generally fits well and feels comfortable, but you still have a little bulging, try a style with a fuller-cut cup to fit fuller shapes of the same size."

Lower the back. The lower the strap fits on your back, the more support you get, says Goldstein. "Wearing a bra strap high on your back will allow your breasts to hang low and give you a frumpy appearance." The lower edge of the band should anchor below your shoulder blades. If the back rides up, the cups may be too small, or the straps may be pulled too tight. The straps should be comfortable, without digging into your shoulders.

Adjust the straps. For the slimmest, youngest appearance, your bra should hold your nipples about 2½ inches below an imaginary line that connects the folds of your underarms. Adjust the straps so that your breasts fall to this point, while the back strap sits slightly lower than the front. "At no point should the straps dig into your shoulders," Goldstein says. "If that happens, but the bra fits otherwise, try one with wider, more padded straps."

Test the band. The center seam of the bra should fall against your breastbone. The band should be snug all the way around, but you should be able to run your finger all the way around beneath it. "Larger women often make the mistake of buying a bra that is supertight because they think that's what they need for support," says Goldstein. "What they end up with is a bra that digs into them all over and gives them very unflattering, heavy-looking lines as they spill out around it. Try larger, wider straps and bands instead of a tighter bra. It'll support you better and make you look slimmer too."

Chapter 24

Age-Proof Your Skin

Following skin-care basics is the only way to keep youthful-looking skin.

Just one unprotected day in the sun irreversibly damages skin cells and DNA. This damage creates wrinkles and age spots, and may lead to skin cancer. That's what a Boston University study found.

It goes to show that while we search for baby-smooth skin in a bottle, something as simple as sun protection truly sustains the promise of youthful skin. Even expensive face-lifts and chemical injections won't help you look younger if you don't take some everyday precautions.

"Do you know what a woman with aging skin who gets a face-lift but doesn't follow the basics looks like? She looks like a woman with aging skin and a face-lift. The basics go a long way," says Barney J. Kenet, M.D., dermatologic surgeon at

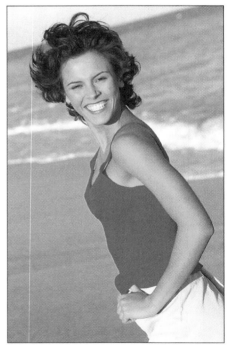

York–Presbyterian Hospital/Weill Medical Center and author of *How to Wash Your Face*. Those basics are sunscreen, sun protection, and a good daily skin-care regimen. They're the keys to keeping your skin youthful and glowing.

There Goes the Sun

Sun damage contributes about 90 percent to the aged appearance of skin. While genetics and aging do play a part in how old you appear, they account for only a small percentage. Most wrinkles, age spots, crow's-feet, sallow skin, blotches, and broken blood vessels come from the sun's rays, not from the aging process itself.

"I have patients who are 80 years old who have beautiful, young skin, all because they stayed out of the sun," says Roger I. Ceilley, M.D., clinical professor of dermatology at the University of Iowa in Iowa City and past president of the American Academy of Dermatology.

You may wonder what the point is in having beautiful skin if you can't bask in the sunshine. You want to be on the beach, on the tennis court, or out in the yard with the kids. Or perhaps you have a job that requires you to spend time in the midday sun. Well, no one is asking you to stay locked up in a dark cellar while the rest of the world romps in the warm sun. You can still enjoy the daylight while protecting your youthful looks, but you must protect yourself with the best anti-aging product on the market: sunscreen.

In fact, the study at Boston University found that using sunscreen every day made patients' skin react as if they hadn't been exposed to the sun at all.

So don't fear if you've spent a good deal of

"Fake It" to Screen Out Rays

It seems that a sunless tan can protect you—a little. Researchers recently found that dihydroxyacetone (DHA), the active ingredient in self-tanners, reacts with skin proteins to produce pigment that screens out UVA, UVB, and visible radiation. Even though it offers an SPF of only 2 or 3, it screens rays that are not blocked by commercial sunscreens. And that extra bit of protection is provided all day since self-tanners resist soap-and-water washing. This is particularly valuable to the very fair-skinned, who burn easily.

Caution: Anyone using self-tanners still needs to use a bona fide sunscreen regularly.

your life running to the sun instead of ducking for cover. Even after years of sunbathing, if you start wearing sunscreen today and every day hereafter, you'll see a marked improvement in the quality of your skin.

"I've seen some remarkable turnaround with just sunscreen. The skin can repair itself to a degree. And because of that, it is never too late to start," Dr. Ceilley says.

Sunscreen: What to Buy

Forget the days when baby oil was the only "sunscreen" you took to the beach. Now, you need a product that offers maximum protection from the sun's rays. The problem isn't where to find it: Just about every drugstore and cosmetics counter is lined with sunscreens and sunblocks in every form imaginable.

What you want is the right sunscreen: one that covers all of your youthful-skin needs. Use the following criteria, and you'll enjoy the sun's rays in peace, knowing you're protected.

Purchase broad-spectrum sunscreens or sunblocks. The sun comes at your skin with two types of rays: UVA and UVB. UVA rays don't make you burn. Instead, they penetrate deep within your skin, resulting in wrinkles and other signs of premature aging. UVB rays burn or tan your skin, producing free radicals, which are molecules that damage skin cells and elastic tissue.

Although both types of rays do their parts in adding years to your skin, UVBs are the most harmful during the summer, while UVA rays bombard your skin all year round.

To fight both UVA and UVB damage, sunscreen should include ingredients such as avobenzone, zinc oxide, or titanium dioxide. But don't worry about remembering highly scientific monikers when perusing the shelves. Simply look for the words "broad-spectrum," Dr. Ceilley says. That means the product blocks both UVA and UVB rays.

Go for SPF 15 or higher. SPF stands for sun protection factor. To calculate how it works, multiply how long it would normally take you to burn by the SPF number. For instance, if

1-MINUTE FAT BURNER

Supersize your H$_2$O. Buy the big bottle when it comes to good-for-you stuff such as water. You'll drink more.

you burn in 10 minutes, an SPF of 15 would allow you 150 minutes in the sun. An SPF of 15 is as low as you can get away with, and it is effective only if you put on a thick enough layer and don't wash or rub it off, Dr. Ceilley says.

If you have fair skin or spend a lot of time out in the sun, wear a product with an SPF of 30. If you have very fair skin or a history of skin cancer, you should use sunblock with an even higher SPF.

Find a double-duty moisturizer. If you're thinking, "Oh great. Another skin product I have to stuff in the medicine cabinet," think again. Many products now combine a sunscreen with a daily moisturizer. Use one to moisturize and protect your skin at the same time, Dr. Ceilley suggests.

Grab some sunscreen lip balm. Your lips need protection from the sun as well. But sunscreen lip balm with an SPF of 15 serves another novel yet practical purpose: Apply the lip balm around your eyes. It won't run or burn when you sweat, and it's easier to apply than lotion or gel.

‖ **Wear It Well**

Choosing the right sunscreen is only half the battle. If you don't use sunblock correctly, your skin still catches all those age-inducing rays. Follow a few simple guidelines, and you'll get the maximum from your sunscreen. Your skin will thank you every time you look in the mirror and don't see a new wrinkle.

Apply 20 minutes before you go out. Sunscreen doesn't give you immediate protection. It takes at least 20 minutes for the active ingredients to soak into your skin. Slather on sunscreen first thing in the morning to ensure that it has enough time to work, Dr. Ceilley says.

Don't be stingy. If your bottle of sunscreen lasts a year or so, you're not using enough. For full-body protection, use 1 ounce, or one shot glass full of sunscreen, Dr. Ceilley says. When applying it just to your face, use a marble-sized amount, he adds.

A recent study found that most people use only 50 percent of the recommended amount of sunscreen, which means that they are receiving only half of the SPF. So if you put on an SPF 15 but don't use enough, it's the same as if you used a sunscreen with an SPF 8. A study at Dryburn Hospital in England found that people who didn't put on the recommended amount of sunscreen received only 20 to 50 percent of the SPF protection on the label. While their bottles of sunscreen may have lasted longer, they wasted their youthful looks.

Reapply. A study at the Queensland Institute of Medical Research in Australia found that reapplying sunscreen every few hours offered 2½ times better protection from UV rays than a single application. If you're working out, sweating, swimming, or doing anything strenuous, reapply every 2 hours. Even waterproof sunscreens eventually wear off, Dr. Ceilley says.

Wear it on all days and in all seasons. Clouds do not protect you from UV rays.

Cold, blustery winter days do not protect you from UV rays. As long as the sun is in the sky—even if you can't see it—those rays will break through and into your skin. Make sunscreen a daily and a yearlong habit, Dr. Ceilley says.

Added Protection

Sunscreen is powerful, but it's just one part of a skin protection program. The rest is up to you. "There is much more that you can do to protect yourself," Dr. Ceilley says. Here's how.

Stay out of the midday sun. You don't need to shun the sun like a vampire during the day. But be conscious of how much time you spend outside between the hours of 10:00 A.M. and 4:00 P.M., when the sun's rays are the strongest. Take a break in the shade, or go inside every hour or so, Dr. Ceilley says.

Wear a hat. A fashionable hat will not only make you look younger but also will keep those skin-ravaging rays away from your face and neck alto-

If you put on an **SPF 15** but don't **use enough**, it's the same as if you used a sunscreen with an **SPF 8**.

gether. Sport a hat with at least a 4-inch brim that goes all around your head. It should completely cover your ears and the back of your neck, Dr. Ceilley says.

Shade the glare. The sun's rays have been shown to promote cataracts, another sign of aging. But on top of that, squinting exacerbates crow's-feet and other lines around the eyes, Dr. Ceilley says. Put on sunglasses with UV protection when in the sun.

Cover up with clothes. When possible, wear long-sleeved shirts and pants, Dr. Ceilley says.

The Fountains of Youth

If Ponce de León were around today, he wouldn't have to travel halfway around the world in search of the mythical fountain of youth. A quick hop to the local mall would be as far as he would have to go to hear tales of magic potions and waters that reverse the marks of time.

But even today, finding a true fountain of youth could prove just as elusive as Ponce de León's ancient quest. While countless ads claim that they have the true youth serum, only two products have been scientifically shown to help erase some of the signs of time such as wrinkles, lines, and age spots, says Leslie Baumann, M.D., director of cosmetic dermatology and assistant professor of clinical dermatology at the University of Miami. Here's how they work and how to use them.

Alpha Hydroxy Acids

As far as over-the-counter anti-aging ingredients go, alpha hydroxy acids (also known by the "eu-

Your Daily Skin-Care Routine

When it comes to daily skin care, keep it simple, says Barney J. Kenet, M.D., dermatologic surgeon at New York–Presbyterian Hospital/Weill Cornell Medical Center and author of *How to Wash Your Face*. Instead of convincing patients that they need an arsenal of skin-care products, Dr. Kenet says that people only need two or three.

Not only that, but how—and how often—you wash your skin can be as important as what you use. "Many people overwash. That dries out skin, making it itchy, flaky, and rough, which doesn't look too nice," Dr. Kenet says.

Follow this basic daily skin-care program and watch your skin regain its youthful glow.

Morning: Body

• Take a 2- to 3-minute shower. Using cool to room-temperature water, get wet, then step out of the shower stream. Lather yourself up with a mild soap such as Dove, Basis, or Cetaphil.

• Stay out of the water stream as much as possible. Do not use loofahs or abrasive washcloths that will scratch and dry out your skin. Rinse off and step out of the shower, Dr. Kenet says. Pat your skin dry with a towel.

• Moisturize your body while your skin is still damp, so that the moisture is trapped. For full-body moisturizers, Dr. Kenet says inexpensive products work just as well as expensive ones, and if you're really on a budget, even olive oil and vegetable shortening can do the job. He suggests avoiding heavily fragrant moisturizers.

• Apply a sunscreen with an SPF of 15 to the areas that will be exposed.

Morning: Face

• If you are just washing your face, use a soap-free cleanser such as Cetaphil Gentle Skin Cleanser for dry skin, or Neutrogena Oil-Free Acne Wash for oily skin. Regular soap may dry out your skin and accentuate wrinkles.

• Dampen your face with tepid water. Apply a quarter-size amount of the cleanser evenly to your face and massage gently with your fingertips. Rinse with tepid water and then pat dry.

• Apply an SPF 15 sunscreen to your face every day. Use a combination sunscreen and moisturizer to save a step in the process.

• You usually would use Retin-A or an AHA product at night, but if you are using both, apply your AHA in the morning. Just be sure to check with your dermatologist first.

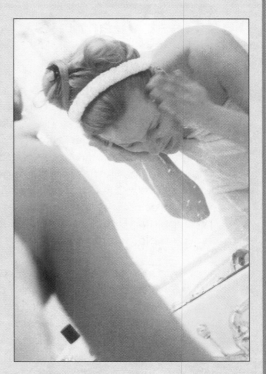

Night: Face

• If you have dry skin, you may not need to wash your face every night, Dr. Kenet says. Excessive washing will dry it out even further.

• If you decide to wash your face, use the same technique you did for your morning wash.

• Apply either an AHA or a Retin-A or Renova product at night, but wait at least 10 minutes or so after you've used a cleanser. Moisture on your skin can dilute the effects of the AHA product.

The Best Vitamin C Skin Care

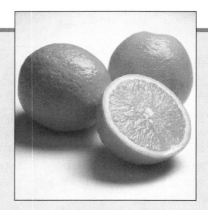

In the correct amounts and in the right formulation, vitamin C (ascorbic acid) can stimulate collagen and elastin production, firming skin and eliminating fine lines and wrinkles. This antioxidant powerhouse also lightens skin, reduces blemishes and brown spots, and protects against future sun damage. Unfortunately, vitamin C is often no longer active in skin-care products by the time you get them home—or it may not have been present in an effective form to begin with. But research has found the formula for stable, effective vitamin C—and cosmetic companies are taking note.

In a recent Duke University Medical Center study, researchers at the Durham, North Carolina, school found that vitamin C is best absorbed into the skin when delivered in a 20-percent concentration of L-ascorbic acid at a low pH. Based on this research, at least one company has already revised its vitamin C formula. The product called Primacy Serum 20 isn't a prescription drug, but is available only through skin-care professionals. To locate a supplier near you, call (800) 811-1660. Other companies are bound to introduce similar treatments. Check products carefully for L-ascorbic acid concentration and pH levels. Don't assume that a higher concentration of L-ascorbic acid is better: Oddly enough, the Duke study found that 25- and 30-percent solutions were significantly less effective.

reka"-sounding initials AHA) reign supreme. These natural acids, the most popular of which is glycolic acid, make you look younger in several ways.

They increase exfoliation of the skin, accelerating the removal of the outer layer of skin to reveal smoother, softer skin. They moisturize, helping to diminish the appearance of fine lines and soften dry, sun-damaged skin. And in higher concentrations, AHAs increase the thickness of the skin's second layer, called the dermis, which gives skin its youthful, glowing, healthy look.

But not all AHA products are created equal. Depending on the product, the amount of AHA varies and will have different results. For instance, one study compared a product with 5 percent glycolic acid to one containing 12 percent. While the 5-percent product did improve the skin's surface, the 12-percent concentration had more dramatic results.

Research has suggested that you need at least a 10-percent AHA concentration to stimulate the formation of collagen, which could help restore a youthful appearance. Although it may improve the smoothness of your skin, an over-the-counter product with a concentration of less than 10 percent won't help to erase lines or wrinkles.

There are a few over-the-counter AHA products (Alpha-Hydrox and Aqua Glycolic are two) that do have a concentration of 10 percent glycolic acid. But most contain less than 10 percent.

What should you do? Start with an over-the-counter product with a 10-percent concentration. Keep in mind that you may need to use it for a few weeks to a few months to see results. If it doesn't work, or if you've had a lot of sun exposure, talk to your dermatologist, who can prescribe treatments with a much higher concentration, Dr. Kenet says.

Retin-A and Renova

Retin-A and Renova are prescription drugs that contain tretinoin, a derivative of vitamin A. You'll have to make a trip to your dermatologist's office if you want them. It may be well-worth the visit: In various studies, Retin-A reversed sun damage, increased collagen formation, improved fine and coarse wrinkling, erased age spots, and evened out skin discoloration.

Retin-A was and still is an acne treatment. After dermatologists noticed its youth-promoting effects, they prescribed it for aging skin. Its sister product, Renova, was created solely for the purpose of treating wrinkles and aging skin. Follow the directions carefully, and ask your dermatologist how these may interact with the other skin products you use.

You can find over-the-counter products containing retinol, another by-product of vitamin A. But no evidence shows that it works as well as its prescription siblings, Dr. Kenet says.

If you want to start with an over-the-counter brand first, give it a try, Dr. Baumann says. If you don't see any improvement, ask your doctor for a prescription for Retin-A or Renova.

Household Items That Double as Beautifiers

Whether you're preparing for a big night out or celebrating a night in, it's nice to know that if you don't keep mud wraps and facial masks in stock, you can just head for the refrigerator or pantry. These suitable substitutes, suggested in the booklet *Instant Beauty* by Memphis herbalist Ray Gailes, can do the trick.

Cat litter. Many cat litters are plain old clay,

Research has suggested that you need at least a 10-percent AHA concentration to stimulate formation of collagen, which could help restore a youthful appearance.

which you can use to make an oil-absorbing mud mask. Mix 2 tablespoons of clean, pure, and 100 percent natural (no deodorizers) clay litter with 1 ounce of water. Mash into a smooth paste. Apply and wait 15 minutes. Rinse.

Lemons and powdered milk. The natural AHAs found in lemons and powdered milk can slough off dry, rough skin and help reduce blemishes and fine lines. Mix the juice of three lemons with 1 cup of powdered milk until a paste forms. Rub on your elbows, knees, and feet. Wait 15 to 20 minutes, then scrub off with a sponge.

Yogurt and honey. Both yogurt and honey contain the AHAs that smooth skin, clean pores, and banish breakouts. Besides being antibacterial, honey holds in moisture. Mix 2 tablespoons of plain yogurt with 1 teaspoon of honey. Apply and wait 5 minutes. Rinse.

Cucumber and avocado. Together, cucumber (with its vitamin A–type compound) and avocado (with its antioxidants) can soothe irritated skin, unclog pores, and help smooth fine lines. Peel, de-seed, and chop one-half of a cucumber and one avocado; and mash them into a paste. Apply, leave it on for 15 to 60 minutes, then rinse.

Vinegar. Use vinegar to reduce acne breakouts by removing excess oil, killing bacteria, and normalizing your skin's pH. Mix 1 ounce of vinegar with 10 ounces of water. Dab on with a cotton ball; allow your skin to air-dry.

Chapter 25

Shape Up
Your Smile

Anyone can have more attractive teeth— in months or sometimes in minutes.

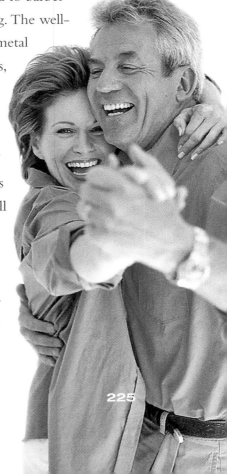

Dazzling white teeth aren't just a modern obsession. As early as the 14th century, Europeans eagerly flocked to barber–surgeons for a crude form of enamel bleaching. The well–meaning quacks filed the patients' teeth with a coarse metal instrument. Then they dabbed each tooth with aqua fortis, a solution of highly corrosive nitric acid.

This procedure did whiten the teeth, at least for a while. But the harsh acid so thoroughly destroyed the tooth enamel that most people developed mouthfuls of painful cavities within a few years. Despite its obvious drawbacks, acid cleaning continued to be popular well into the 1700s.

Nearly 300 years later, dentistry has developed much safer and far less painful ways to satisfy the quest for brighter smiles. The following tips and modern-day treatments can help anyone who is dissatisfied with the look of her smile.

225

23 Reasons to Smile

If you were blessed with straight white teeth and healthy gums, all you need to enhance your smile is to do it more often. But for the rest of us—and one in two Americans rank themselves among the dentally dissatisfied—these simple tricks and cutting-edge treatments will come as welcome news. Nowadays anyone can have more attractive teeth, sometimes in months, sometimes in minutes. Here's how.

1. To make yellowish teeth instantly look whiter, use a lipstick with a bit of blue in it, says makeup guru Laura Mercier. Blue turns up in a surprising range of shades, from cool red to pinky brown. Don't be put off if a color looks purplish in the tube; test it on your lips, preferably in natural light. Avoid any hint of copper or orange.

2. If your teeth are gray, try a warm tone of lipstick such as coral or rose. Just don't pick a shade that's too blue or yellow.

3. Check out the latest at-home bleaching kits available from your dentist. Some require only an hour of wear a day for a couple of weeks, so you can leave the mouth guard on while you're doing chores or watching TV instead of while you sleep. This method can lighten surface stains three shades. The $400 to $500 cost includes extra gel for touch-ups.

4. For more stubborn stains, including the type sometimes caused by taking tetracycline, ask your dentist about "power" bleaching. The technique uses lasers or other sources of very bright light and heat to activate a highly concentrated peroxide gel. And it offers instant gratification: white teeth in just an hour or two. Expect to pay $900 to $1,500.

5. Don't assume that you have to tolerate those smile-dimming metal fillings. New and improved ceramic materials are almost invisible, and they're less sensitive than metal to heat and cold, says Miami dentist Gordon Sokoloff. Your insurance may even cover some of the replacement cost.

6. A straw isn't just for slurping watered-down diet soda from the bottom of a paper cup. It can keep stain-causing liquids from touching your teeth. Use one to sip dark juice, cola, or tea—especially the reddish fruity kinds, which are among the worst tooth tarnishers.

7. Keeping stains at bay is even simpler when you drink coffee or hot tea: Just add milk.

8. Cracked, peeling lips accentuate stains and prominent gums *and* make your mouth look older. Exfoliate regularly with a washcloth, toothbrush, or the Body Shop's Lipscuff, advises San Francisco makeup artist Tana Emmolo Smith. Moisturize at night with Elizabeth Arden Eight-Hour Cream (the version in the lipstick tube), petroleum jelly, or lip balm.

9. De-emphasize a gummy smile with a neutral lipstick just a shade darker than your mouth, suggests New York makeup artist Paula Dorf. Skip anything that grabs attention, like a shimmer.

1-MINUTE FAT BURNER

Pay cash for treats. Anytime someone offers you goodies—and you accept—put $1.00 aside. Then give the money to your kids. When you literally pay for treats, you're more likely to say, "No, thanks."

Sensitive Teeth

The enamel shell that covers your teeth is the hardest substance in your body, providing a protective coating that shields the nerves in your teeth as you chew. Should this protective coating wear off, any hot or cold temperature can trigger pain, says Kimberly Harms, D.D.S., a dentist in Minnesota and consumer educator for the American Dental Association. You know you have sensitive teeth if you bite into a Popsicle and your teeth immediately send a bolt of pain to the center of your brain.

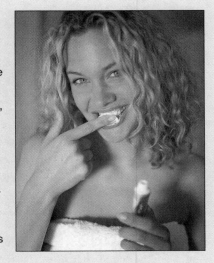

"The more you can do to preserve the enamel coating, the better," says Dr. Harms. "Otherwise, you start having problems." Here's how to help keep your teeth hard and strong.

Go softly. Use a soft toothbrush, and don't brush too hard. Bearing down on your teeth can wear away the enamel, particularly near the gum line, where it's not quite as thick.

Brush in a circular motion. The tips of the bristles should gently clean slightly below the gum line.The next time you go to the dentist, show the hygienist how you're brushing, to be sure you're doing it right.

Floss daily to remove plaque. If allowed to accumulate, a sticky film of bacteria-laden dental plaque can prompt your gums to pull back a little. Since enamel covers your teeth only down to the gum line, the newly exposed tooth will be more sensitive.

Buy toothpaste for sensitive teeth. Widely available at supermarkets and pharmacies, these toothpastes contain substances that build up on the surface of your teeth like an artificial coating of enamel. Be patient; you may need to use the paste for several weeks before you notice any improvement.

Talk to the expert. Let your dentist know whenever your teeth hurt. If necessary, she may be able to seal them with a protective coating. And if you have just one tooth that is extremely sensitive, visit your dentist right away—the problem could be a damaged nerve, which calls for immediate treatment.

If you wake up in the morning with clenched or tired facial muscles, you're grinding your teeth in your sleep and don't know it. Your dentist can fit you with a mouth guard to protect your teeth from further damage.

Don't Make This Mistake

Chewing ice is extremely rough on your teeth. Not only can it wear away enamel, it can actually crack your teeth, exposing the sensitive dentin (the principal tooth material below the enamel) to the food, water, and air in your mouth. If you think you may have cracked a tooth, see your dentist right away.

10. Fix prominent gums permanently by having a dentist sculpt them (usually the gum line is adjusted) so your teeth look longer. New diode lasers quickly cauterize tissue so there's little pain or bleeding, says Richard Hansen, who teaches at the Center for Esthetic Dentistry at the University of California, Los Angeles. The procedure, known as crown lengthening, costs $1,600 to $1,800.

11. Don't let stress wear down your smile. About 25 percent of people grind their teeth, usually while asleep and often without knowing it. This is damaging to front teeth as well as molars. If you wake with a sore jaw or other facial pain, or you notice loosened teeth, consult your dentist, who can fit you with a mouth guard.

12. Let a computer show you how you'd look with straighter, shapelier teeth. Many dentists now offer custom smile design at no cost. So does the American Association of Orthodontists; for information about getting a free computer-generated photo, write to Smiles, American Association of Orthodontists, 401 North Linbergh Boulevard, St. Louis, MO 63141.

13. If your front teeth are slightly crowded or your incisors would do Dracula proud, the solution may be as simple as filing away a bit of enamel. Reshaping, or enamel contouring, is quick and almost painless; the cost is $75 to $100 per tooth.

14. A gap that's more Alfred E. Newman than Lauren Hutton can often be fixed with bonding. An enamel-like material (usually a plastic called composite resin) is painted onto teeth, sculpted, hardened, and polished, all in an hour or two. The cost is $300 to $700 a tooth.

15. Check out high-tech braces. The newest materials, clear acrylic and tooth-colored ceramic, make them nearly invisible. For many adults, targeting a handful of teeth (usually the lower ones, which tend to crowd with age) will work wonders in mere months, says Denver orthodontist Christopher Carpenter, a spokesman for the American Association of Orthodontists. And many dental plans cover at least part of the $1,800 to $4,500 cost.

16. There's an even newer, faster way to straighten your smile: Veneer it. By changing the size, shape, and spacing of a few front teeth, long-wearing translucent wafers of ultrathin porcelain or composite resin can make you look as if you've had years of orthodontic procedures, says New York dentist Robert From. Veneers can even mimic plastic surgery: Applied to side teeth, they fill out a drooping mouth; on front teeth, they plump up sunken lips. Plus, they whiten better than any bleach does. Expect to pay approximately $1,000 per tooth.

17. If your gums are seriously eroded, take heart. Thanks to advances like lasers and imitation skin, it's easier, quicker, and less painful than ever to cover exposed roots so that teeth are prettier and healthier. Insurance may cover some of

HealthPoint

Hormone Therapy Can Save Your Smile

If you're weighing the pros and cons of hormone-replacement therapy (HRT), add another entry to the list of pros: HRT may slow the progression of gum diseases, the number one cause of tooth loss in people age 35 and older. These diseases trigger inflammation that can destroy both the gum tissue and the underlying bone that holds teeth in place.

In a study of 70 postmenopausal women being treated for gum diseases, those who had lost bone mass and were on HRT had less gum inflammation and lost less supporting bone than those not taking HRT. Although most of the women on HRT took a combination of estrogen and progesterone, it was the estrogen that seemed to do the trick by dampening inflammation, says the lead researcher Richard A. Reinhardt, D.D.S., Ph.D., professor of surgical specialties at the University of Nebraska Medical Center College of Dentistry in Lincoln.

Discuss the benefits and drawbacks of HRT. Let both your doctor and your dentist know if you or anyone in your family has a history of gum disease, osteoporosis, heart disease, breast or colon cancers, or Alzheimer's disease.

Follow the basics of good oral hygiene. See your dentist regularly, floss daily, and brush your teeth at least twice a day.

Don't smoke. Tobacco use can not only lead to bone loss but also make your mouth more vulnerable to bacterial infections.

the $900 to $1,200 cost of the surgery, known as ridge augmentation.

18. Don't assume that a new smile is beyond your budget. Taking a cue from plastic surgeons, many dentists now offer installment plans or arrange "smile loans." To find out more about financing, treatments, or specialists in your area, call the American Academy of Cosmetic Dentistry at (800) 543-9220, or visit their Web site at www.aacd.com.

19. In addition to your regular brushing and flossing, drink lots of water. H_2O stimulates the production of saliva, your mouth's first defense against plaque. Drink even more

as you get older, because saliva output winds down with age.

20. If you've forgotten your toothbrush, chomp an apple, a stick of celery, or a carrot. Crunchy foods get mouth juices flowing, so they're great natural cleansers.

21. Pay extra attention to your gums if you're pregnant. Hormonal changes may predispose mothers-to-be to early-stage gum disease, which can lead to the more severe kind, periodontitis, and has been linked to low birth weight. Birth control pills, which mimic pregnancy, also make some women prone to gum ailments, says Barbara J. Steinberg, D.D.S., a dentist and professor at MCP Hahnemann School of Medicine in Philadelphia.

22. Ditto if osteoporosis, or diabetes runs in your family. Research suggests that people with either ailment have a high rate of severe gum disease.

23. Clean your tongue. It's the best way of beating the more than 200 kinds of odor-producing bacteria that collect there. Use a toothbrush or a plastic scraper, sold at any drugstore. The result will be a breath of fresh air.

LIFESTYLE RESTYLE

Never Too Old to Lose

Connie Bissonnette had all but given up on slimming down. At age 50 and 172 pounds, the full-time university instructor from Stillwater, Minnesota, believed that weight gain was a normal part of the aging process.

Lucky for her, her son Jeff knew better. Yes, most of us do gain weight as the years roll by. But this accumulation of extra pounds isn't written in our genes. We may blame weight gain on our hormones or the laws of nature, but the most likely bottom line is simply that we spend too much time lingering in our recliners instead of walking around the track.

In 1992, Jeff was a student at the University of Wisconsin, majoring in human performance. When he came home for Christmas break that year, he had a mission: to persuade his mom to start exercising. "I was his first project," Bissonnette jokes. And as a result of his persistence, she's 41 pounds thinner.

She responded with her usual litany of excuses: she didn't have time, she didn't have the energy, her knees bothered her. But Jeff persisted. "He said, 'Just give me 10 minutes three times a week,'" Bissonnette recalls. "He devised a workout that I could do at home, with what I had on hand. I started out by sitting in a chair and doing leg lifts. Then I added other exercises, like doing pushups against the wall."

Despite her initial protests, Bissonnette found herself enjoying her workout. Within a few months, she noticed that her knees felt better. So she asked Jeff to add some more exercises to her routine. Her 10-minute exercise sessions stretched to as long as 30 minutes. Plus, she started walking for 30 minutes, 2 or 3 days a week. One year later, she was 20 pounds lighter.

But Jeff wasn't done. His next challenge was to transform his mother's longtime meat-and-potatoes diet. Again, he advised Bissonnette to start small. She substituted jam for butter on her morning toast, fresh fruit for her snack-time potato chips and candy bars. Eventually, she traded frying for baking as her cooking method of choice.

It took some time, but all those little changes added up. Four years after she began exercising, Bissonnette had lost a total of 41 pounds. Now age 58, she has maintained her weight at about 131 pounds since 1996.

Bissonnette was so grateful to her son for helping her slim down that she decided to return the favor. In May 1997, she became a certified personal trainer. Now she works in her son's gym. "It's great to be able to encourage the clients I train by telling them about my own weight-loss experience," she reports. "I don't let anyone say, 'I can't.'"

Credits

"What We Really Eat" on page 14 is adapted from "Food Pyramid: Ideal vs. Real" © 2000 by Consumers Union of the United States, Inc., Yonkers, NY 10703-1057, a nonprofit organization. Reprinted with permission from the March 2000 issue of *Consumer Reports on Health* for educational purposes only. No commercial use or photocopying permitted. To subscribe, call (800) 234-2188 or visit us at www.ConsumerReports.org.

"Are You Strong to the Core," "Your Upper-Body Oomph," and "Can You Shop 'til You Drop?" on pages 81, 83, and 84 are adapted from "The Physical Fitness Specialist Protocol for Muscular Endurance Testing," a training manual from The Cooper Institute for Aerobics Research. © 1999 by the Cooper Institute for Aerobics Research. Reprinted with permission.

"Am I Too Sick to Exercise?" on page 91 is adapted from an article of the same name by Myatt Murphy that originally appeared in *Self*. © 1999 by Myatt Murphy. Reprinted with permission of the author.

"Health Problems? Shape Up the Right Way" on page 92 is adapted from "Shaping Up: Workouts for Special Disorders" © 2000 by Consumers Union of the United States, Inc., Yonkers, NY 10703-1057, a nonprofit orga-

nization. Reprinted with permission from the January 2000 issue of *Consumer Reports* for educational purposes only. No commercial use or photocopying permitted. To subscribe, call (800) 234-2188 or visit us at www.ConsumerReports.org.

"Why Your Size Matters" on page 109 is adapted from an article of the same name by Myatt Murphy that originally appeared in *Self*. © 1999 by Myatt Murphy. Reprinted with permission of the author.

Cover photograph

© by Hilmar (newsstand edition only)

Interior photographs

All interior photographs by Hilmar except those listed below.

Eyewire: page 2

© by Brian Hagiwara: pages 44, 45, 46

John Hamel/Rodale Images: pages 86, 97, 168, 202

© by Sam Jones/Outline: page 159

© by Graham Kuhn: page 227

Mitch Mandel/Rodale Images: pages 41, 56, 57, 167, 191, 222

Rodale Images: pages 146, 199, 184

© by David Roth: page 214

© by John Sterling Ruth: page 153

© by Tony Stone Images/Hutton Grey: page 110

Kurt Wilson/Rodale Images: pages 47, 65, 66, 67, 68, 70, 73, 74, 75, 76, 83, 120, 164, 189, 198, 200, 221

INDEX

Boldface page references indicate photographs.
Underscored page references indicate boxed text.

A

B